PRAISE FOR AGING POWERFULLY

"While thoroughly practical, *Aging Pow...* chronicle of one woman's life told in detail. The central focus is health, especially in one's golden years (the seventies and beyond). There are many antidotes in terms of diet, exercise, mindfulness, and spirituality. Having gone through turbulent times with an eating disorder, the author is well poised to offer some real advice. After all, she had knowledge of the human condition from inside and out.

The well-written and example laden content is a guidebook for others, using herself as the prime example. There is no more powerful way to convey the intended message. It is factual, well researched and compelling. Anyone who faces life's many challenges, especially as they age, will find something here to identify with.

In short, it is a life laid bare in order to help and save others the grief of suffering an addiction that is altering the very substance of one's life. It ends with encouragement and easy-to-follow guidelines that are sure to change the readers' perspectives, most profoundly on the subject of aging."

~ Carol Kay, Author

"Your book is remarkable in its practical insights and wisdom, and it's clear that you have done considerable research in writing it. The most important aspect of any book is its substantive content—and you have great content. You're offering your readers wonderful, substantive information that can enrich their lives considerably (I'm now going to look into the plant-based diet for me and my family!).

The book is also clearly written and logically presented. There are no issues of incoherence of a lack of consistency. In other words, the structure and organization is also very well done.

I want to reiterate what an amazing project this is, and I know it will encourage and inspire your readers. Your insight and wisdom, coupled with your vulnerability, is truly remarkable."

~ Renee Skiles, Writer

"As someone who has struggled with an unhealthy relationship with food for most of my life, Nan's book gives me hope. Through the power of story, *Aging Powerfully* offers real, practical, well-researched tools for reclaiming power in their own lives. Part memoir, part self-help guide, the reader is given an inside view of how a pattern of disordered eating can develop, and how it can be disrupted. By aging p.o.w.e.r.f.u.l.l.y., Nan lays out a roadmap of positive lifestyle modifications that can have long-lasting and life-changing effects. The journey is yours to take."

~ Cati Porter, Author

AGING POWERFULLY

Accept Your Past and Take Control of Your Future!

Find Vibrant Health, Balance, and Joy with

NAN SIMONSEN

Certified Integrative Nutrition Health Coach

Plant-Based Nutritional certification from eCornell University

Specializing in Lifestyle as Medicine

Aging Powerfully
Accepting your past and taking control of your future
Nan Simonsen

The content of this book is for general instruction only. Each person's physical and emotional condition is unique. The instruction in this book is not intended to replace or interrupt the reader's relationship with a physician or other professional. Please consult your doctor for matters pertaining to your specific health and diet.

Printed in the United States of America

ISBN-10: 1-7363310-0-0
ISBN-13: 978-1-7363310-0-2

I dedicate this to all who have known the feeling of being powerless, whether young and incapable of taking control, or at any point in adulthood, when it becomes clear that there is need for a change.

My wish for us all is to fully grasp that we have the power within us to alter the direction of our health, and therefore our life. I dedicate this book, and the rest of my life, to taking command of what we can, and *AGING POWERFULLY!*

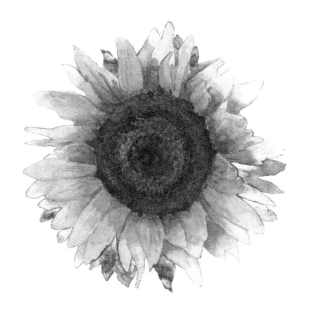

THE SUNFLOWER
helianthus annuus

Wherever life plants you,
bloom with grace.

~ Old French proverb

We each have a particular flower that informs our soul. For me, it is the sunflower. When I imagine, see, or hold a sunflower, it lights me up on the inside. It brings a smile to my face, and energizes my step. Why? It is not the most beautiful of flowers. It is neither colorful, intricate, delicate, or fragrant. It doesn't necessarily play well with others. In a vase it can be a bit brutish in this way. Why does the sunflower speak so deeply to me?

First and foremost, because the sunflower is tough. It has to be. It springs up from the poorest of soils. It represents resilience under undesirable circumstances. In human terms, as I see it, that translates to strength, confidence, tenacity, flexibility, faith, focus, optimism, and longevity. The sunflower has been held in high regard for thousands of years and seen by some as a spiritual flower which bespeaks true faith, loyalty to something bigger and brighter than oneself, self-respect, and authenticity. These are all traits that I admire.

To the traditional Chinese, the sunflower characterizes long life and good luck, even for a time to be eaten only by royalty to insure immortality. Its yellow color signifies vitality and intelligence. For the Chinese, the flower is a symbol of happiness and joy.

In Native American symbolism, the sunflower is used in late summer festivals as a symbol of bounty, harvest, and provision. It exemplifies the sun, and is thus likened to the life-giving force of the Great Spirit. The color is noted for its vitality and embodies energy as well as fertility.

I don't think there's anything on this planet
that more trumpets life than the sunflower.
For me, that's because of the reason behind its name.
Not because it looks like the sun,
but because it follows the sun.
During the course of the day,
the head tracks the journey of the sun across the sky.
A satellite dish for sunshine.
Wherever light is, no matter how weak,
these flowers will find it.
And that's such an admirable thing.
Such a lesson in life.

~ Dame Helen Lydia Mirren

CONTENTS:

ACKNOWLEDGMENTS

With deepest gratitude to Amie Olson, my art director and publishing agent, for her time, patience, attention to detail, and remarkable abilities. I could not have completed this project without her, nor would I feel the pride of accomplishment without having had her skillful intervention.

Thank you Carla Bender, my brilliant photographer, who brought out the best in me.

Thank you to my dear friend Anja O'Kane who stepped up immediately after I began writing my manuscript to offer a second set of eyes. She did far more than that with her clever and creative recommendations.

Thank you to my long-time friend (and my jewelry designer) Jennifer Katz, for being with me both when Bob passed, and as I was writing, checking in along the way.

Thank you fellow Master Gardener, Lucy Heyming, and her husband Frank Heyming, for offering their magnificent five-acre garden property, and cathedral-like, newly rebuilt redwood barn, for my January 9 birthday and book launch celebration. As a writer herself, Lucy was the first to review my initial work and to tell me that yes, I could write. She also gave wonderfully insightful recommendations.

Thanks to my dear son Erik, for taking the time (twenty minutes before leaving for your five day beach-front vacation) to brainstorm the appropriate words for the subtitle for *Aging Powerfully*. So much to say; so many ways to say it. You nailed it honey!

Thank you to my two talented and generous editors who not only allowed me to write in my flow of consciousness style, but allowed me to look good while doing it. Both also kindly offered to review my book:

Carol Kay was given everything that I wrote in the first pass, made sense of it, and helped to clarify my words into legible passages. She is an accomplished writer.

Renee Skiles skillfully reviewed the finished project by sections, astutely made corrections, and then reviewed the finished manuscript before and after it was formatted into book form.

Thank you, Cati Porter, for your offer to read my manuscript and to review it. A brilliant writer with nine books of your own, your evaluation is invaluable.

Thank you Dr. Wayne Dysinger, staff and patients for welcoming me into your Lifestyle Medical practice as an Integrative Nutrition Health Coach. My view of health has been formed and cemented by my involvement with your practice. It is also with humble gratitude that I extend my sincerest thank you to Dr. Dysinger for the beautifully written Forward that he contributed to this book.

To the men in my life: My dear Bob who loved me in spite of all he knew and who believed in me until the end. We had 40 great years together. And to my dear husband Tim for your support and patience during the demanding process of writing this book. What a joy to have you in my life. Grow old along with me, the best is yet to be!

FOREWORD

Aging Powerfully begins with a hard but real story. This is followed by a transformation that was both a battle and a gift. It finishes with an inspiring challenge that is surrounded by opportunity. It's the story of one life, and of everyone's life.

Each person's story is their own. In this book Nan is honest and vulnerable telling her unique and compelling story. It is those same qualities that empower her call for revolution – not just within herself, but within all of us. And its that concept, moving from the individual to the community, that is the promise of *Aging Powerfully*.

I've worked with Nan now for two years. She is the real deal. Her knowledge is immense and hard won. Her experience is broad and nurtured from real life. Her heart is deep and embracing of all. This book is sharing that person not just to individual patients and groups, as she does in our practice, but to the whole world. I'm proud of her, and of this book.

I recommend *Aging Powerfully* to anyone who appreciates real stories, desires genuine transformation, and aspires to a long and healthy life. Prepare to have your heart pulled, your mind challenged, and your world inspired. Lifestyle Medicine offers the potential for a healthy life to 90 or 100 years of age for all who choose it. Nan shows you how she overcame difficulties and is claiming this promise for herself. You can too, for yourself, your family and your community.

Wayne S. Dysinger, MD, MPH
Physician, Founder and Chair, Lifestyle Medical
Cofounder and past president of the College of Lifestyle Medicine

INTRODUCTION

We age, and then we die. We cannot control these, but to a great degree, we can influence them. The current trend is that this scenario is happening at a younger and younger age.

Join me as we buck the trend.

Let's live vibrant, balanced and joyful lives.

Together, we can AGE POWERFULLY!

Imagine living into your senior years, surrounded by friends who are equally as vibrant and engaged, enthusiastically envisioning the next year, five years, one or more decades. You had that fire in your gut in younger years, so let's bring it back again!

I wrote this book because I have seen first-hand, and experienced personally, how energetic we can feel, and therefore how vivaciously we can live, when we adopt simple evidence-based lifestyle habits. Now in my 70s I am more excited about the possibilities in these next twenty to thirty years than at any time in my life. Let me share with you why and how, and take you with me on a mission to age with power. Let's create a movement to encourage others to do the same.

Taking control of our health and how we age, knowing that we have the ability to orchestrate the outcome, is a liberating experience. What about genetics? Our genetics may load the gun, but our epigenetics (our behaviors and environment) pulls the trigger. More than 80% of our ultimate health outcomes are based on epigenetics. So again, we have the power.

Aging Powerfully will take you on a road trip. The story that I tell helps put into perspective all that follows.

- In Part 1, *The Past,* my health journey is put into context when I relate the progression of formative years that affected me deeply, nearly destroying me, and then positively forming me. I will highlight as I go, the lessons learned.

- Part 2, *Taking Control,* offers the roadmap to what becomes the science and evidence-based fundamentals of health that I offer. This discussion will help you to take control of your health and, ultimately, the way you will experience life.

- Part 3, *Aging P.O.W.E.R.F.U.L.L.Y,* and 4, *Living F.U.L.L.Y,* will offer what you need to move forward with enthusiasm and eager anticipation to the transformation that will take place as you evolve toward your mission to age powerfully.

When you finish this little book, you will have the inspiration, the direction, the resources, and most importantly the vision of what life can be when you embrace that vision and make the commitment to age powerfully.

As I explain in this book, approaching my 70th birthday gave me pause. There is no way around it, 70 is considered old age. As an Integrative Nutrition Health Coach, working under one of the founding physicians of the College of Lifestyle Medicine, with patients in our Lifestyle Medical family practice clinic, I was able to see first-hand the power that a patient has to heal themself when given the instruction and support to embrace the concept of lifestyle as medicine. Hippocrates, the father of modern medicine, said nearly 2,500 years ago that our body will heal itself if given what it needs. He added "Let food be they medicine, and medicine be thy food." Yes, it is as simple as that. Let me show you how.

When you finish *Aging Powerfully*, my desire for you is that you can clearly and with steadfast determination direct your actions toward bucking all current trends of chronic disease in America and join my mission to set an example. My desire is to convince all who will listen, that there is a far better way to age. A way of aging that leads to a rewarding and passion-filled life, rather than one of slow, sad, physical and emotional degradation. Again, I say, join me. Be with me on this mission. Let's show what growing into our older years can look like and relish in every day as we do it. "Grow old along with me. The best is yet to be!"

PART 1:
CHALLENGES

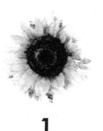

1

THE POWER OF PARENTING SETTING THE GROUNDWORK

Parenting: noun, a father or mother; verb,
be or act as a father or mother to (someone).

Ellen Perkins, author and empowerment expert, wrote, "Without a doubt, the number one most psychologically damaging thing you can say to a child is 'I don't love you' or 'You were a mistake.'"

Setting the Stage

It was late winter, 1954. The sanctuary of St Catherine Laboure Church in Torrance, California, felt familiar, yet overly majestic and frightening. We three children were dressed for Sunday service, although it was mid-week. We were so young, innocent, and vulnerable. Edgardo was two years old; I was three, and Stephano (Steve) was four. My mother must have been devasted as we walked into the church; her heart and mind shattered into a million pieces. We lived just a few blocks from the church, and we had walked there. Today I now wonder how my mother had managed to deal with that day.

A nun welcomed us into the church. Our shoes echoed through the never-ending marble hallway. She led us to the office of a black-robed priest. I don't remember his words, but I very clearly recall their meaning. Our father would not be coming home to live with us ever again. We all cried.

My perception at the time: Our father no longer loved us.

My fair-hair, blue-eyed father, who immigrated from Naples, Italy, in 1946, married my mother, a black-haired, olive-eyed, first-generation Italian, from a far less illustrious family. Together they had three children. Ultimately, he became bored with my mother, who, he later told me, "became too fat and unkept." Through her pain and shame, my mother revealed to us that Dad had another family with whom he was now living. Life became very hard for my simple, emotionally damaged mother. When she was very angry, she would accuse us of having driven our father away.

My perception at the time: 1) To be worthy of love, you must be thin; and 2) We had been replaced by better children. We were a mistake.

In the mid-fifties, all our friends had present and engaged fathers. The black and white television shows at the time featured loving functioning families, with stay-at-home mothers and happy, well-adjusted children. My mother's status as a divorced woman brought her shame that seeped into our consciousness. She could no longer attend Sunday mass due to Catholic restrictions, so we were brought by a friend, or we simply didn't go.

There was little to no money. At times we couldn't afford food. The humiliation still burns as I recall the repeated scene of standing at the counter of our neighborhood market while the kindly Asian grocer handed me a bag of the cheapest meats, canned goods, and wilted produce, writing our name on the receipt and slipping it into the register. We would pay it when we could manage. It is with the utmost gratitude that I remember the grocer, as well as the elementary school teachers who exhibited empathy and compassion toward us three children, desperately in need of additional direction. During those years, from kindergarten through the eighth grade, we attended the same school, just one block from our apartment. With after-school programs, the staff helped raise us.

Parenting matters. Lessons learned, perceived or otherwise, often color our view of the world and of ourselves. My mother was dealt a lousy hand of cards. Her dreams had been crushed, her self-esteem shattered, and her existence became a perpetual struggle. Unfortunately, she was not at all equipped to deal with these challenges.

At the end of the eighth grade, she moved us to Poplar Bluff, Missouri, with one of our neighbors from Torrance, an alcoholic, whom she had married. He not only abused us verbally, especially Steve, but he physically abused Mom. We literally escaped with nothing but a bag of things when a teacher from our high school offered to take us to an out of town bus station the night the police took him away for putting a gun to my mother's head. Since he was a "hometown boy" and we were the crazy Californians, he was released from jail the very next day. Thank God we were gone.

From age fourteen to seventeen, I attended high school in Yucaipa, California. In the mid-sixties, it was a one-offramp town an hour east of Los Angeles. My mother's parents ran a small hotel there, and Mom would help with the paperwork and maintenance. After our year of terror in Missouri, my life-battered mother had somewhat checked out as a parent. By then she had bonded almost exclusively with Steve, my artistic, sensitive, damaged, and compliant older brother, leaving Edgardo and me to our own devices. Deep emotional troubles shadowed each of us. Drugs—LSD, methedrine, and marijuana—helped, and then hurt, as we tried to navigate through those pivotal years.

Help! Get Me Out of Here!

My first suicide attempt was during my sixteenth year. During a family visit, my beloved grandmother glared at me and yelled in broken English that my mother had told her I was ruining the family. She pointed her crooked finger at me and said, "You're no good!" My only remaining emotional safety net, the love and closeness of my Nanna, had unraveled. Upon returning home, I locked myself in the bathroom and took a full bottle of Steve's Thorazine (prescribed for depression and mood disorder). I climbed out of the bathroom window and ran until the drug kicked in and dulled my senses. In a grassy field, I laid down, expecting to die. Little did I know then that an overdose of Thorazine doesn't kill you. At least, I didn't die. It was nighttime when I woke up, dazed and disoriented. Mom had called the police, and they had found me wandering in the dark. They escorted me home, and no one acknowledged or ever spoke of this again. Water under the proverbial bridge.

My perception at the time: I'm in this on my own—so toughen up.

There were other methods to bypass emotional pain. Depending on our temperament and personality, we make our own choices, and I soon found another method to deal with the pain. Although some people dull feelings with drugs, alcohol, shopping, sex, and any number of destructive behaviors, I outsourced my emotions to food. Food: the use and abuse of it.

I was always a skinny kid. When I began to fill out in my mid-teens, my mother, perhaps feeling the need to stem the chubbiness that had haunted her, pointed out that I was getting heavier. Remembering my early lessons regarding conditional love, I simply stopped eating. That worked until, at eighty-something pounds, I passed out in gym class and was told to eat or be hospitalized. My brother Steve, who was at that time into bodybuilding, confessed that in order to stay "ripped," he ate and threw up. And then he told me how.

With no sense of true north in any area of my life, I grasped at yet another straw so I wouldn't drown in the muddy waters of my emotional world. I was off and running as a bulimic. How could I have known that this disorder—this addictive behavior, with all the stress, shame, and personal degradation in tow—would haunt and control me, off and on, for more than fifty years? How could I have known that I would hold onto it for most of my adult life?

My perception at the time: Food was my best friend, but also, food was my nemesis and could be my worst nightmare.

Time to Move On

It was 1967. I was sixteen. My car, a little blue Corvair, was T-boned and totaled by a sedan that ran a stop sign. The collision caused the car to spin and slam into a tree. My only injury was a knee laceration from the gear shift knob, which required a trip to the emergency room and a litany of the line "You are so lucky!" from the attending staff. The thunderous sound, and the jolt of the dual impact, have not left me, nor has the scar.

After the accident, the $700 insurance check (a lot of money in 1967) was one month late, and then two. When I called the insurance company, I was told that it had been mailed. When I asked my mother, she informed me that it hadn't arrived. A full-time summer babysitting job bought my car, and I had no money for another. Betrayal, fury, and personal diminishment echoed inside me when, with yet another call regarding my wayward insurance check, the representative confirmed that my mother's signature was on the back of the check, dated sixty days prior. Mom had lied to me again. She had not only received it, but she cashed it. Mom used the money to purchase equipment for Steve's newly-formed musical group. My car and the money were gone. That was the day when I realized that I had to leave home.

Our Family Disintegrated

Edgardo quit high school at age fifteen. A bully beat him up at school. The principal did not hesitate to point out that Edgardo's long hair naturally attracted "this kind of negative attention" and directed that he cut it or not return to school. That was his last day of high school. He moved in with a friend's family in Benedict Canyon, an area in the southeast of Los Angeles. Years later, he finished his GED and went on to earn two graduate degrees, one in music composition and another in orchestration. He has orchestrated many Hollywood movies, the best known being the *Men in Black* series.

Steve graduated from high school and moved to Hollywood to play his music. Being both musical and artistic, he later created art for Hanna Barbara Productions. Mom followed him, renting them an apartment together.

Like my family, the crowd I was running with in Yucaipa, California, scattered. After two drug busts, a sixteen-year-old friend becoming pregnant, and an overdose leading to death, my crowd was falling apart. The local police labeled me "one of them," but actually, I wasn't. I didn't like alcohol, I had smoked marijuana only twice, and I experienced only two acid trips, both of which terrified me. I considered these people my friends because they accepted me; I had no others. The few things I owned were packed, and I left home at the end of my junior year of high school.

My perception at the time: I had nothing to lose because I had nothing.

Home and Still Alone

How does one redirect their life? By changing the things that influence one's actions. My father, who we seldom saw, lived with his wife and two children, who were just a few years younger than his first brood, in West Los Angeles. He ran a thriving contemporary art gallery, a sprawling indoor/outdoor extension of rooms and courtyards built onto an old home in a business district. Whether he offered or I asked, I can't remember, but I moved into a storage room in my father's art gallery. One way or another, in the summer of 1968, at seventeen, I left behind the tough chic person that I had become, sans heavy makeup and car, and I went to be with my father.

His wife wanted me away from the well-bred children, and, except for a few meals together, I spent very little time outside my room. It was clear that I wasn't welcome, and I told myself that I didn't belong in his world. With no "good" clothes and, by his assessment, overweight (128 at 5'2"), I didn't "validate" my father, who preferred I stayed in my room when important clients visited the gallery.

Shame permeated my self-assessment throughout my senior year at my third high school. I left my old life behind. I no longer desired any part of it. But simultaneously, I had no guideposts to reinvent myself. I had no friends, and I was kept separated most of the time from my father's "proper" family. I struggled to read and comprehend math. Four decades later, when I returned to college for a landscape design certification, I was finally tested and diagnosed with ADHD and dyslexia.

Alone, in a back room of an art gallery, without heat or air (bad for art), I took solace in food. Internalizing emotions—uncertainty, fear, loneliness, and self-loathing—was too hard. Food quickly became my best friend, my entertainment, and the devil. I would binge and purge, sometimes in a day-long trance-like state, just to make it through.

Eating disorders are known to begin in times of self-imposed restriction. Mine began at age fourteen with anorexia, which transitioned to bulimia, ultimately becoming entrenched as my way to deal with emotions— both good and bad. I now understand that anxiety and depression accompanied me like a looming cloud during this lonely time.

My perception then: There was nothing else I could do to ameliorate the pain.

A Second Attempt

It was a cold and cloudy winter morning in 1969—a school day. I was eighteen and a few months away from graduating from high school. What I remember about my second suicide attempt was the shroud of near manic depression that enveloped me. My life and circumstances had become intolerable. I had absolutely no one to talk to. I felt ugly, fat, and unwanted. I hated myself on so many levels, including stealing money out of my father's change box to go to the corner liquor store for binge food, gorging on the food, and then struggling painfully to bring the food back up. I had to escape. Leaving my purse, shoes, and glasses behind, I boarded a 5:50 am bus to the beach, paying with a handful of change. When I got there, it was dawn and rather peaceful, without a soul around. In a haze, I walked across the sand and into the surf. I began to swim through the waves, one after another, out to sea. Ending my life was the only way out of my misery.

They found me. But how? Who notified them? To this day I still don't know.

Wet and in a cell, a Coast Guard representative calmly explained that their boat had pulled me from the water and that my family was there to take me home. When I walked into the small room, sitting at the steel desk in the middle of the room, both my father and step-mother began to yell, "How could you do this to us?!" They were relentless and asked it again and again. My feeble response was that I was sorry, followed by my explanation, through tears of shame, that I could not stop eating and vomiting. There was little conversation after that. They left me in my room at the gallery and went back to their proper lives.

After that ill-fated, albeit fortuitous, attempt to end my life, in a dismal abyss, this event and the reasons behind it were never again spoken of with my family. They made it clear that I had done them a disservice, that I was ungrateful and unworthy of having been taken in. Explaining my desperation surrounding my disgusting binge-purge behavior, they shunned the subject. My need to escape who and what I had become was of no interest. Taking me in was unfavorable and clearly more than they had bargained for.

My class graduated in June of 1969. I had no friends, and my family had no interest in my life. So, I skipped the graduation ceremony and received my diploma by mail. That summer I worked as a receptionist in a medical office, and I began Santa Monica City College in the fall.

My perception at the time: *Your pain and problems are YOURS. Deal with them.*

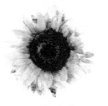

2

THE POWER OF DISORDERED EATING

Bulimia nervosa was first described as a variant of anorexia in 1979 by British psychiatrist Gerald Russell. Historically, references regarding over-eating and vomiting go back before the well-known Roman and Greek vomitorium.

The "system" now had me on its radar. Having been registered by the Coast Guard as a near-drowning/suicide, a social worker sought me out to arrange counseling through the end of the school year and summer. With $75 a month to live on, I could not pay for a therapist, and my father, who did not believe in them, would not have offered. The Coast Guard literally saved my life. The therapists figuratively did the same. I didn't need to die to be saved, I simply needed to be heard.

Meeting with a counselor meant that I no longer had to bear my burden alone, as if my binging/purging were a secret hidden in an emotional black box. But most of those whom I met were unfamiliar with binge-purge behavior. A cringe-worthy memory still leaves me feeling small. A nice-looking, youngish male therapist asked me to bring food along to our appointment, to eat in front of him. As I did so, I felt like a freak being examined by a gawker, hoping for a thrill. I was afraid that I might have disappointed him. I ate without drooling. I swallowed without disgorging. I finished without incident. To this day (as I remember it), I wonder what spectacle he thought he would witness.

Another therapist asked questions that allowed me to put into words the cold space I held deep within: my perception of the unworthy, unwanted, broken little girl who did ugly things that she could not stop. Things that made her forever unlovable. Things for which she felt terrible shame.

A Glimpse of Hope

Overeaters Anonymous held its first meeting in Hollywood, California, in January 1960. These meetings were and still are based on a 12-step program, fashioned after alcoholics and gamblers anonymous. A woman named Rozanne S., who suffered from addictive behavior toward food, noticed similarities between other addictions and her own behavior. As a result, she launched the organization with this first meeting. By the time a counselor advised me to attend, they had been meeting for nine years. I felt that I had finally found a home where I was understood and, more importantly, accepted for who I was.

The meetings were held in the poorly-lit basement of a church. Participants were weighed and given a food plan. There were no bulimics in this group, and at eighteen, I was the youngest there, but the addictive behavior and the obsession with food were identical. Despite the 45-minute bus ride to the church (how fortuitous that it was even this close), I attended three or more times per week for several years. Overeaters Anonymous, with its 12-step program, helped me regain my dignity and self-esteem. I was as sick as my secret, but I no longer felt the scourge of it. I made meaningful connections, my "disgusting" behaviors could be spoken of, and judgment was left at the door. Many people found complete recovery in those rooms, although I didn't. I owned the books, I said the words, and I worked the steps, but I never completely walked the walk.

Round and Round We Go

What followed, as it relates to my disordered eating, was, sadly, nearly fifty years of exactly that, on-again and off-again recovery. I repeatedly dealt with secrecy, shame, aberrant behavior, untold damage to my health, and thousands of otherwise valuable hours lost, hours in which I could have truly lived and enriched my life. And this is not to mention the money wasted on food that was never meant to nourish my body. Sorrow, worry, stress, tension, anxiety, loneliness, insecurity, fear, fatigue, boredom, deprivation, and failure were all trigger emotions—as were happiness, success, and celebration. Each and every one of these emotions, unpredictably, could precipitate a deep dive into a feeding frenzy, and then, because of my early training to avoid weight gain at any cost, a purge. Although, at times, it required more effort, as the illness progressed, I could typically bring up food by simply contracting my stomach muscles.

Because bulimics can consume anywhere from 1,200-10,000 calories in one day, and because purging does not completely empty the stomach, many still have weight issues. My father was heavy-set, and he later died suddenly at sixty-two of a heart attack. His father had faced the same at fifty-nine and his mother at sixty-one; both were overweight. Perhaps it is possible that he was projecting his fears onto me. The end result was a lifetime of weight obsession. My self-worth, and the intensity of my food-obsessed thoughts, were based on the numbers on the scale; needless to say, I weighed myself daily. I was either only good or bad. Worthy or unworthy. Restricting that day or a bit more relaxed.

There were endless recovery efforts and countless therapists applying innumerable modalities. I went back to Overeaters Anonymous many times and for years at a time. Weight Watchers worked again and again. But the obsession would return, and the binging was its consequence. There were many long periods of remission from my food addiction, as it is now referred to medically. And yes, it had all the qualities of an addiction. Substitute the word "food" for "drugs" or "alcohol," and there was little to no difference in my lack of power to control my behavior.

What follows classically describes any addiction: I could not stop. When a triggering emotion, situation, or event occurred, the urge took my control. This destructive binge-purge behavior interfered tremendously with other activities. I planned my whereabouts around food. I put schemes in place to obtain goodies for the next binge so that execution was just a matter of a few easy steps. I would go to any length to binge, regardless of how risky the behavior. The quantities of food consumed could be enormous. I would mold my behavior and routine to accommodate a binge.

Secrecy was crucial. No one but my late husband ever knew. I didn't hesitate to spend huge amounts of money on binge food, although I am generally rather frugal. I vowed every day (during the time I was binging) that I would quit. With all my might, I meant it until one of the emotional triggers would become too unsettling. Urges would become too pronounced. Whatever rules I was following at the time were only there to be broken, little by little. Slips would begin to occur. Then a binge and a purge, and I was again caught up in the painful madness that was my biggest abomination. But I helplessly relived the cycle over and over. I was utterly out of control. Hating who and what I was. A blanket of shame covering all that I accomplished. I was pretending and meticulously trying to look the part of a woman who was in complete control—cool, confident, secure, professional, even admirable. Fooling everyone, including myself, until I could find something to stop the vicious cycle again. At least for a while.

Disordered eating led to discomfort around food—actually, a fear of food. To be more precise, disordered eating led to a fear of my behavior around food. This led to a half of a century of struggle, off and on. I never knew when a trigger would be tripped, and I would dive headfirst into irrational thoughts and behavior around food. There was no enjoyment in a binge. Perhaps joy only in anticipation. Maybe the first few bites. Then came the rationale, and any semblance of eating for pleasure took a back seat to obsession. I was trapped in an almost punishing cadence of shoveling food in and purging it out, all in secret. No one could know or my image of confident self-containment would be shattered. Regardless of the price I had to pay, I would not allow that to happen. Despite hundreds of therapy sessions, my disordered relationship with food persisted.

If I had learned then what I know now, then my days could have been so much brighter and more meaningful. My life would have been far richer, more peaceful, serene, engaging, and connected. But I sacrificed these blessings for food.

Ultimately, loving myself, believing in my worth, honoring my intuition, calming my mind, and trusting myself to make good decisions helped me overcome my need to take comfort in food and to embrace the reality that my life was safe, satisfying, and manageable without regular periods of zoning out and numbing with food.

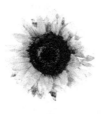

3

THE POWER OF LOVE

Love [agape in the biblical Greek] is patient and kind;
love is not envious or boastful or arrogant or rude.
It does not insist on its own way; it is not irritable or resentful;
it does not rejoice in wrongdoing, but rejoices in the truth.
Love never ends.

(1 Cor. 13:4-8a)

Love changed *everything*. Well, not everything. As stated before, one of the most enjoyable parts of life, for the majority of people—eating and sharing meals with others—remained an on-again, off-again struggle until my mid-sixties. Love allowed me to flourish in spite of this handicap of my own making.

Love, consideration, caring. What may be considered a casual conversation by one person may give hope and direction to another. This knowledge colors my interactions with people to this day. I was in my father's gallery, near closing. I felt and looked like a nobody. Mrs. Krummer, a regular client, entered through the main door, having come to pick up a piece of art she had bought directly from the artist's show brochure. It was late, and with the gallery empty, I was out of my room and sitting on the steps that led down to the main showroom. Mrs. Krummer asked if I would permit her to sit with me. At first, I felt uncomfortable, but she quickly engaged me in a simple conversation.

This tall, slim, elegant lady with silver hair pulled back in a sleek bun, with her Rolls Royce in front of the gallery door, was speaking with me as if I were somebody. Before she stood to go up into the office, she said to me, "You know, Fernanda (my full name), you are smart; you can be anything you make up your mind to be." That was precisely fifty-five years ago. Her name and her elegance are rooted in my head, but her words and how she made me feel are deeply engraved in my heart. *She left me feeling that maybe, just maybe,* I could be somebody.

Dr. Chew, my biology professor during my first year at Santa Monica City College, quickly noticed that I enjoyed the subject. Although reading was a struggle for me, I paid careful attention to her lectures and later asked her relevant questions. She also holds an important place in my memory and heart because I felt valued when she asked me if I would consider being her office and lab assistant. Working alongside such an intelligent woman for a year, being respectfully engaged in conversations with her, and given guidance as if I was somebody made me feel that I was. While I still felt too insecure to make friends in class, as her assistant, I built self-esteem and felt valued. Perhaps I had something to offer.

My first year in college I spent hiding in the back of every classroom. It was in English literature class, during my first semester, that I shared the back row with a quiet, tall, good-looking blond with bright blue eyes. Neither one of us dared to take the first introductory step, so we sat silently next to each other for the first two weeks of class. Then one day he asked if I had finished the assignment due the following week. Oh, no!

Although ADHD and dyslexia would not be recognized for decades, and I thought that I was defective, I tried mightily to keep up with my assignments, but the pattern kept repeating itself throughout my education. I would fall further and further behind as the class progressed. I read poorly, and solving word problems was nearly impossible. Numbers were an enormous challenge, and formulas were utterly overwhelming. At times, the stress surrounding this pattern led to binges, sometimes even during school hours, as desperation and anxiety set in.

Going back to the assignment, I was caught off guard when he asked if I had finished it. With no time to think of a lie, I simply said no. Those blue eyes were on me when he asked if he could help. Although I realized that it would become clear how far behind I was, I agreed. That is how it began.

His name was Bob. He was 6'2", and he towered over my 5'2" frame. He had been a Marine sergeant in Vietnam, and he had been discharged two months prior. Later I would find out that he had been shot in the head during one of the bloodiest battles of the Vietnam war, the 1968 Tet Offensive, losing three-quarters of his platoon while in the hospital. This naturally affected him for the rest of his life. We both had scars. We both had secrets.

A few weeks later we drove to Santa Monica Beach to meet his mother and father. Bob picked me up in his shiny new metallic blue Mustang, which he had gifted to himself after saving most of his military pay. When I walked into the house, his mother excitedly exclaimed, "It's YOU!" It was clear that the surprise was just as pleasant for her as it was for me. Dorothy was a nurse at the medical office at which I worked during the summer. Before I left to go to school, she had given me Bob's photo (which I immediately lost), asking me to say hello to her son who was returning home from the war. In other words, I was already pre-approved. Once again, I found love and acceptance. My self-worth was growing.

Bob and I got married the following December in 1970. He was twenty-three, and I was nineteen. He loved me unconditionally throughout our marriage. He recognized my worth rather than focusing on my faults. His acceptance and love became the cornerstone of my self-esteem. At that time, he saved me.

In spite of the handicap that my challenges with food posed, Bob and I made a good life together. In college I studied food and nutrition. Bob studied civil engineering as an undergrad, and later he successfully completed a graduate degree in public administration, all while working full-time. In 1970, he began his career and quickly rose in status in the Department of Public Works for the City of Los Angeles. As for me, after starting in the business office of Santa Monica Hospital, I was promoted to dietary supervisor. I became familiar with the workings of a commercial cafeteria, as well as patient dietary preparations.

We purchased our first home in 1972 and moved to the San Fernando Valley, a suburb of Los Angeles. The move required that both of us commute to work, unfortunately in opposite directions. During our first six years, we decided not to have children. In my case, I feared raising a child, not sure that I could trust myself to stay present and focused on a baby's needs rather than my own addictive behavior. As it played out, in January of 1977, I was pregnant. Having read health expert Adelle Davis' *Let's Eat Right to Keep Fit*, I kept my eating during the pregnancy clean and controlled. Erik was born on his due date, after a two-and-a-half-hour natural drug-fee delivery. He was healthy and beautiful.

Being home full-time with a young child gave me too much unstructured time. I could see the signs that I was slipping back into disordered eating. Four months after Erik was born, I was easily persuaded to join a Tupperware sales team by a lady doing a friend's demonstration. I liked the product, and I knew food preparation, storage, and my way around a kitchen. Bob was fine with me taking off after dinner to do in-home demonstrations, leaving him to put Erik to bed. Little did either of us know that the innocuous decision to take up a simple part-time job would lead to a twenty-eight year highly successful and fulfilling career in direct sales.

More importantly, the leaders of the Tupperware company that I was so fortunate to join, Sylvia and Jon Boyd, became two of the most influential people in our lives. Brilliant, beautiful, and talented, Sylvia became my role model in business and in life. She recognized my skill sets and coaxed me to develop heretofore under-appreciated abilities, all the while applauding my growth. To this day she, and Jon are like family to me. I quickly built a team of consultants and realized that I had the ability to teach, train, and inspire people as a team leader. Within five months, I earned a company car and the pride and influence it offered.

Bob took care of what I struggled with due to my learning disabilities, such as filling out orders correctly and general paperwork. Seven years later, in 1985, Bob left his stable, secure, and very well-paid job as a LA City Superintendent to open a Tupperware franchise with me fifty miles east of Los Angeles, in Riverside, California, also known as 'The City of Trees'. It became the talk of Los Angeles City Hall that this high-ranking civil engineer was quitting and leaving his lucrative pension plan and benefits package to sell plastic. We had the last laugh. Throughout the years spent working together, we shared the satisfaction of building a multi-million-dollar-a-year business in our pretty little university town. We ran it for twenty years and had a great time doing it. We found comfort in the knowledge that we had plenty to retire on.

During our final ten years in Tupperware, we enjoyed life in a 4,000 square foot dream house, on 2.25 acres. Shortly after moving in, we enrolled in a one-year, University of California-sponsored program to become certified Master Gardeners. Our goal was to create a botanic garden on our two-plus acres. Within three years of taking ownership of our mostly-barren property, we were featured twice in Sunset Magazine and opened our home to garden tours and events for seven consecutive years.

After retiring from Tupperware, I studied landscape design to gain the skill of rendering a plan. I then enjoyed fifteen years as the owner of Nanscapes, my landscape design business. During that time, I created more than 220 water-wise gardens, winning many environmental design awards. During this time, Bob chose to fulfill a lifelong goal of writing. After retirement, he began to write the first of what would become three military books. He also re-engaged with Vietnam-era Marines from his battalion. Life was good to both of us.

The Good Life, But Still Addicted

In my late fifties, I was happy, satisfied, and confident in who I was. And yet, in spite of that, I continued to struggle immensely with my eating disorder. Even then, no one but Bob knew that I was bulimic. Therapists, medications, dietary plans—nothing helped me to heal fully. Much later, and especially now, I realized that, at least for me, I was going about recovery the wrong way. Although it has been quoted again and again, "It's not what you're eating, but what is eating you." My addictive behavior was present regardless of my frame of mind. Settling with past demons became the focal point of therapists during sessions but, in the end, did not play a part in my recovery.

I treated my body poorly when binging. However, due to my obsession with health and nutrition, I chose a healthy diet—lean meats, legumes, whole grains, and masses of vegetables and fruits—mainly home-cooked. This saved me health-wise. All disordered eating disrupts and damages the body, anorexia and bulimia, especially so.

But I don't underestimate the steep price I paid psychologically. I was weighed down by an emotional shroud for more than fifty years due to this secret, the shame I felt, and the knowledge that I wasn't who and what people thought I was. All forms of hiding and dodging our demons carry a high price. With deep gratitude, as I write this, I am describing life in the past, no longer in the present. I have been free for more than two years and have no fear of going back. It would no longer be acceptable, and I now have the tools that will allow me to continue to reject it. More on this later.

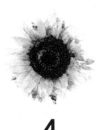

4

THE POWER OF ACCEPTANCE AND LOSS

Erik's phone was ringing. I was praying that he was available to talk. Still in shock, my mind was racing. It wasn't supposed to go this way. The date was Friday, November 26, 2009, the day after Thanksgiving. During our holiday meal, the family had given thanks, believing that Bob was in recovery, while asking for the strength to see us through the expected upcoming surgery.

We were at the Veteran's Administration Hospital in Loma Linda, California, to set the date. With the goal of enabling Bob to eat more comfortably again, we were anticipating an esophageal resection—not an easy procedure, but manageable. Upon initially entering the exam room with Bob, Dr. Wallens' demeanor instantly caused me to catch my breath. The words that followed punched the tiny remainder of air right out of me. "I am so sorry to tell you this, Bob, but the cancer has metastasized. It is now in your lungs and liver. The chemotherapy and radiation did not work."

Bob was physically broken after two months of grueling chemotherapy and radiation. His throat and esophagus were in shreds. The cool green smoothies that our brand-new, high-end power blender whisked together to nourish him no longer slid down his mangled tube. Dr. Wallens reiterated that his stage 4 esophageal cancer was now metastatic, explaining the ramifications. We were advised that the treatment he had been given was the most advanced available and that there were some "experimental" treatments that could be attempted. However, Bob refused to go any further. He was too ravaged and in too much pain.

After this devastating news, Bob calmly asked, "How much time do I have?" Understandably, the doctor deferred, not wanting to be that direct. My Vietnam hardened Marine wasn't having it. "How much time do I have?" "You have four to six months," the doctor replied. Bob's quiet response was, "During the Tet Offensive of May 1968, on the day I was shot in the head and presumed dead, two-thirds of my company were killed. Since then I have strongly believed that I was on borrowed time. I will now join my brothers, who lost their lives that day." He then added, "I will die at home. No more treatment!"

While home hospice was being arranged to begin that Monday, Dr. Wallens kindly offered to come in the following day, a Saturday, to insert a stent into Bob's esophagus to prevent potential collapse and widen it to allow food to pass more easily. While they discussed the details, I left the room to call Erik.

Erik, now thirty-two and our only child, picked up the phone, thinking that I was calling with the date of the surgery. Leaning against the cold wall inside the hospital restroom, surrounded by nothing other than institutional green, I wept as I told him that his father would not recover and was dying.

Embracing Reality

Accepting hospice care meant the end of additional horrendous procedures and their side effects, forgoing the anguish of disappointing expectations and false hopes, as well as the mitigation of the severe pain that had plagued him constantly. It also meant that during the time he had left, instead of fighting the reality, we embraced every day we had together as a gift. We spent our precious time connecting more meaningfully, talking, playing games. We took daily walks until he became too unsteady due to the drugs. Humor dies last and will power never dies, so we switched to a wheelchair, continuing to cover two miles nearly every morning, getting coffee at a 7-Eleven along the way. It was decent enough coffee, but more importantly, it was a destination nearby. And rituals mattered. We went out to lunch daily to those restaurants that could happily accommodate Bob's particular requirements—pureed food. We were so grateful for the waitresses' kindness and the repeated willingness on the part of the busy cooks to fuss over his food. Most lunches lasted a couple of hours. Time was spent eating, talking, and playing cards. Leisurely, lovingly, even happily.

Happily. That is how I remember it as I write ten years later. The journal that I kept at the time, which I pulled out and dusted off in order to be clear on a few details, has shined a light on a dusky corner of my suppressed memories.

> Today, the writing becomes about the reality of this unfolding ghastly year. This morning, at 2:00 am, Bob woke up gagging from stomach acid, then threw up blood—dark brown and grainy. What this tells me about the progression of his disease is jarring. At times, he says his pain is unbearable. More methadone and morphine were then supplied.

> This year must be dedicated to shoring up reserves emotionally, learning to cope with fears, considering how to move forward with grace and dignity. I jauntily followed with a favorite euphemism, 'Ladies, gird your loins,' from the movie The Devil Wears Prada.

> It is early morning. I have lain in bed for hours crying, feeling the pain of the impending loss of all that we are. Forty years! Shit!!! I feel hollow, dark, frightened, so lonely and purposeless. In advance of this coming reality—brittle, exposed and abandoned.

In spite of these expressions, accepting what was coming made every moment more poignant. As people say, at times casually, "We are all going to die sometime." The last word of that pronouncement is the catch. With the near proximity of that date and the clarity that each season is one's last, one can rail against the gods in fury or accept and even embrace the crystal-clear understanding of one's mortality. We chose to do the latter.

Doing it Our Way

Bob had already retired when he was first diagnosed with stage 3 esophageal cancer in July 2009. My business, Nanscapes, was flourishing, and I had three active landscape designs due, with multiple clients booked for consultations. Within a few weeks, I finished the pending designs but informed everyone on my waiting list that I was suspending my business to be with my ill husband. Bob's involvement in several community projects was canceled, and word got out that his cancer was terminal.

Brave Laurie Lucas, a writer for our local paper, the *Press Enterprise,* heard about Bob's diagnosis and asked if she could write an article about us. Interestingly, it didn't strike us as offensive or intrusive, and we agreed. The article was beautifully written and focused on how a local businessman and published author was spending his final months. It was comforting to speak with Laurie and express how strongly we felt about the control we could still exercise over our lives. Our goal was to create meaning.

Unexpected people stepped forward to offer acts of kindness. For example, a prayer shawl was knitted by the prayer group of a neighbor I had never before met. It was cathartic to be able to speak openly of this most profound and impactful event. Acceptance was a blessing we gave each other, and in an interesting way, to others.

On Saturday, December 19th, less than three weeks after our world was rocked by Dr. Wallens' prediction, Bob and I hosted the wedding of our son, Erik, to our daughter-in-law, Dina, at Riverside's historic and elegant Mission Inn. Erik and Dina, who lived in Jacksonville, Florida, had announced their engagement to one another in September, knowing that time was of the essence. They choose the Saturday before Christmas for their wedding, in order to coordinate it with their holiday visit.

Serendipitously, Bob and I were also married a Saturday, December 19th. We celebrated our 39th and final anniversary on the date of Erik and Dina's wedding. Mystical and magical. Bob's condition was known by all, and although this wedding was a triumphant celebration of Erik and Dina's new union, it was an especially beautiful moment when Bob and I were asked to take the floor for our final anniversary dance.

A Life Grows, Another Fades

Erik and Dina contacted us at the end of January with the exciting news that they were expecting a baby. The due date was the third week of September. If he could hang in there, Bob would be a grandfather. More news in April—Erik accepted a position in Mumbai, India, and they were moving in late May. Before they left, we were given a 4D sonogram of our grandson "Luke" in utero, moving, stretching, and holding his umbilical cord. I was amazed at this technology—the sonogram video was set to soft background music. By then, Bob had lost more than fifty pounds and was wheelchair-bound, but I believe that sonogram and his longing desire to meet his grandson, if not in person but via Skype, extended his life by months.

Grandpa Bob missed Luke's birth by seven weeks. As I write this, Luke just celebrated his 10th birthday. He dearly loves his PapaPapa, has his military memorabilia in his room and is fascinated by stories relating to the Marine Corps.

My Bob accepted his impending death with dignity and grace. The increasing dosages of morphine to help dull the pain interfered with him finishing his third military book and led to prolonged hours of sleep, but he never complained. He spent a good deal of time "training me" so that I would be able to cope with the tasks that he had happily taken care of throughout our marriage—managing our finances, paying bills, balancing checkbooks, and so much more. He reminded me that we always paid charge card bills monthly, and running up debts was a bad practice. Fortunately, four years before, we had downsized from our large dream house to a quaint eighty-year-old cottage in a historic district of the city, for which we paid cash. We were completely debt-free, a situation that I have since maintained. He wrote page after page of loving instructions. When the shaking of his hands hampered his writing, we switched to him dictating as I wrote.

Up to the point of Bob's illness, I had dealt with my emotions, my highs and lows, feeling peaceful or stressed, by turning to food. At times, I couldn't wait to be alone with some otherwise forbidden food and get lost in the ritual that was to follow. There couldn't have been a more emotionally-wrought period in my life than during Bob's illness, his death, and my learning to go through my days without him. My initial fear was that we would both decline together: Bob from esophageal cancer and me from bulimia. Nothing in my past would have led me to believe that anything else was possible.

Within weeks of coming to grips with his impending death, however, I realized that I was not using food as an emotional crutch as I had done previously. There was no binging. No purging. There was no comfort taken in the kitchen while Bob slept upstairs. My disordered eating, obsession with food, and inability to relieve stress without getting lost in mounds of junk food all disappeared within a couple of weeks of our being told that he was terminal. A life-long escape hatch was suddenly, willingly, slammed shut. For *five years,* my eating disorder disappeared.

I was nineteen and Bob was twenty-three when we married. He died at sixty-two. I was fifty-nine. During his final months, the question of who I was without him haunted me. Forty years together. Although I launched and ran two successful businesses, he took care of anything and everything that I couldn't, which was a lot, especially all business-related matters involving numbers, which were impossible for me to keep straight. He made me look good and appear capable. I loved him even more for never judging me and for the beautiful soft spot that he held for me in his heart.

As I am writing this, I notice the date, July 24. Bob died on July 24, 2010. Ten years ago today he died at home in my arms. It was such a blessing that two dear friends, Gerrie Brewington, whom I had known for over 30 years, and Jennifer Katz, also the designer of the silver jewelry that I pridefully wear, were there with us and for us. As Bob was taking his last breaths, Jennifer read Robert Frost to him, and when he was gone, she helped release his soul. As Bob's soul separated from his body, a part of mine escaped with it.

Our hospice worker came soon afterward, and all of us raised a glass of wine in Bob's honor.

My mind's eye examines these ten years since Bob's passing, and I feel proud of the strength that I have mustered, the lessons that I have accepted and learned, the person I have become, and the confident and tenacious woman who looks back at herself in the mirror. Bob would be impressed and proud. Some say he knows.

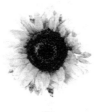

5

THE POWER OF MOVING FORWARD

A Change of Scenery

Even with seven months to prepare for his death, Bob's passing hit me hard. I was devastated and numb. Getting him through his final months had become our project, and our bond became even stronger. When he was gone, I was dumbfounded. Wait, what happened? Where did he go? When would he give me "a sign," as he had promised? Not having a deep religious conviction, there wasn't anything that I could hold onto. He was just gone. Gone. I remember feeling completely alone. Not lonely, but alone. Vulnerable. Fragile.

More than 350 people kindly joined me at Riverside National Cemetery for Bob's memorial. Nearly 200 came to the house afterward to celebrate his life. Such generosity of spirit! Nevertheless, I felt encased in a bubble—separate from it all. Three days later I flew back to Mumbai, India, with Erik, who had returned home to lay his father to rest. I would be with him and Dina for the birth of my beautiful grandson, Luke, who was born less than a month later.

I would also assist them with the complex details of establishing themselves in a newly built luxury apartment on the 29th floor, in an ex-pat community of Powai; a suburb of Mumbai. They moved in three months after their promised date, well after Luke was born. India is a great country to visit, but a very complicated and challenging place to navigate in daily life. Erik and Dina bravely embarked on their journey of raising Luke there for the first three years of his life.

When I left home for India, I had originally planned to return to California within two months. A reliable in-home pet sitter was hired to stay at the house. Fortunately, she could extend her stay because I would not find my way back home for six months. After Luke was born and they were settled in their new home, I realized that I could best 'find myself' by going out into the world on my own. Using the internet, I booked several consecutive international tours. Occasionally I would give myself a few days in between tours to stay behind and further explore on my own before jumping on another plane to the next destination, most likely in another country.

After returning from my first six months abroad, I continued to travel. In all, I visited fifteen countries in just fifteen months after Bob had passed and saw a lot of the world. During this period, I encountered hundreds of very different people, and I saw myself through the eyes of strangers. I liked what I saw. During my travels, away from everything that once had been so familiar to me, I was confronted with many challenging, uncomfortable situations. I conquered them all—some better than others. I gained a new perspective of myself, my strengths, and my position in the world. I surprised myself since it was all positive. I gained unimaginable confidence in the person I had become. She was brave. Adventurous. Capable. Likable. A survivor. All of this, without once falling back on my old crutch—my nemesis—my eating disorder.

Grief Lingers, But Not Forever

After my six month absence for international travel, and between additional trips, I successfully reactivated my landscape design business, was reinstated on the board of the UC Riverside Botanic Garden and became socially active again. I spent a lot of time with friends and acquaintances, both entertaining and being entertained. In spite of that, a pervasive numbness blanketed me for the first year after Bob's death. My emotions were felt in a very narrow range. Although I wanted to step out of the ordinary and experience all that I could as a newly single person, anticipation, enjoyment, and appreciation were blunted as if my consciousness existed on an alternative plane.

One memorable example was my decision to go skydiving ten months after Bob passed away. I called the facility, which had a last-minute cancellation, and therefore an opening the next day for a tandem dive. I registered and showed up as required one and a half hours early for an orientation and video. Those going up on my flight were all with friends. I was alone. They exhibited either giddy anticipation or outright fear. I felt nothing.

I was assigned an instructor with whom I would be tethered for the tandem jump. As he helped me with my dive gear, he expressed surprise this sixty-year-old fragile looking female was there alone. When the twelve of us boarded our small airplane, and as we climbed to 12,000 feet, and then as we prepared to jump, he asked if I was scared, if I was excited, or if I had questions. My answer to all of his inquires was no. I can still recall how oddly neutral I felt, in spite of this extreme experience. Even after we jumped for the free fall to 7,000 feet and then feeling the jolt and subsequent swing through the air when the chute opened, I still felt nothing. And then, even when we were about to come swooping in for our butt-slide landing, as the ground was rapidly approaching—nothing!

Looking back at this experience, and the photos that were taken during the dive, what I remember most was the sound and the rush of air during the free fall, the beauty and calm of soaring under the open shoot, and the pride I felt for this independent act. It was an allegory for that first year without Bob.

My most pressing desire during the skydiving experience was to share it with Bob. In a way, I did just that. Two months later, one year to the day after his death, I went up again with the same dive instructor, again on a tandem jump. Up in the air, I released Bob's ashes, 7,000 feet above the earth. May your soul be free, Bob.

Looking back at my journal during that period, it is clear that although I had gained confidence in who I was and my ability to navigate life on my own, everything was overshadowed by a deep and heavy sadness. I can't say that I was clinically depressed. I was simply painfully saddened by the loss of my dear partner and the life we shared together. To this day, when the memory of that painful goodbye is stimulated by a similar situation on film, or a spoken by another recounting their story, tears will fall.

Life Goes On

We are regularly reminded that life goes on. I trusted time to perform its magic, and I began to heal. It was nearly imperceptible, but slowly my soul and spirit began to thaw. The cool veil of aloofness that kept people, joy, and engagement at an emotional distance began to wear thin. Pleasure in small things, like spending time in my garden, reveling in the wafting scent of flowers, the experiencing joy watching our resident squirrels surreptitiously gather and hoard seed pods, began to break through the numbness. Although I accepted that Bob was gone, it took that first year to stop looking for signs of communication from him, to accept that his transition from me and this world was actually and fully complete.

The last part of my reawakening became evident when I slowly gave myself permission to entertain the thought of love again; something that he made clear was his wish for me. Having reveled in the warmth of a partner and missing the closeness that a serious relationship offers, I accepted the possibility of a new man in my life. With the help of friends, I ventured out into the scary world of dating. At first it felt awkward, actually wrong on so many levels, to be with another man, in any capacity.

I knew what I wanted and surprisingly met a dear man who checked all of the boxes, and more. He had been divorced for ten years and had raised his two daughters on his own, from ages eleven and twelve, until they were on their own. His name is Tim Kelley. He is a year and a half younger than I am, and he is a CPA and tax attorney. I married him on Saturday, November 24, 2012. With Tim, I not only found a new husband, but I gained two smart and beautiful grown daughters, Kristine and Jackie. Kristine and husband Manny blessed us sixteen months ago with a new grandson. My own grandsons gained a new grandfather, Papa Tim.

Again, It Reared Its Ugly Head

Life was good. Tim and I truly enjoyed each other, and because he owned his own firm and I owned my landscape design business, we could control our schedules, and we began traveling within months of getting married. We took three to five trips annually. The year after we married, Erik and Dina, having moved from India to England, had their second son, Liam, a source of utter delight for them and me—actually, us. Tim thoroughly enjoys the two grandsons, now ten and seven.

Fast forward nearly a decade. The 2020 coronavirus pandemic occurred shortly after we returned in January 2020 from a cruise through the Panama Canal and up the Pacific coast of Costa Rica, putting an end to our travel this year. We are both health-conscious and fit; we enjoy exercising every morning, as well as a thirty-minute brisk walk each evening. During our years together, Tim could never have guessed that I had struggled with an eating disorder, and for our first four years, I felt confident that it was in the past and that I would "take this secret to my grave." Not having fully understood what had triggered the disorder to actually vanish, I was devastated when it returned, fearing that it would take ownership of me again and control me as it once had. I also knew that unlike Bob, Tim would never accept it.

How and why did the binging begin again, after five years of living comfortably free of it? In 2015, Tim was diagnosed with a tumor on his pituitary gland, which is in an area of the skull behind the nose and eyes, surrounded by the brain. This pituitary adenoma, although benign, was pushing on his optic nerve and had to be removed. Although not technically so, the surgery was akin to brain surgery. We were both scared but too scared to admit our fear to one another. If this didn't go well, the Tim going into that surgery room might have been very different from the Tim who came out, that is, if he survived at all.

In a bizarre twist of circumstance, Tim's surgery date was the date of my late husband's death. Neither Tim nor I are religious or superstitious; however, there was an unspoken awareness of this significance as he was taken into the operating room that morning for what was going to be a seven-hour surgery. Could this have been Bob's curse on us, or his protective hand reaching out? That evening, the neurosurgeon, Dr. Clark, reassured me that the procedure had been completed successfully and advised me to go home and rest for the night. Tim was going into the ICU, where he would stay for nearly a week. They let me stay with him, and I didn't leave his side for the following five nights.

My fear and tension were so overwhelmingly strong after Tim was taken into surgery that I had nothing but coffee that day, leaving me totally depleted, both physically and emotionally. On my way home from the hospital, I stopped at a nearby cafe with a salad bar that we both enjoyed. Everything about that day was too much for me. I should have gone home and gone to bed. Instead, I ended up having too much of the salad buffet. I felt stuffed and out of control of everything—the dinner, my emotions, and worst of all, Tim's outcome. The meal became a binge and led to a purge.

Although this time, the disordered eating did not return to the previous level of severity, it came up from time to time and caused me shame, distress, and fear. Fear, because I knew that it would end my marriage; Tim would have no understanding, nor tolerance, of that level of weakness in me. Naturally, I was assuming this, because I had no way of truly knowing. But I believed it to be true, and yet I could not conquer this ugly behavior.

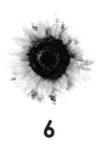

6

THE POWER OF INSIGHT

For emphasis, I will repeat, my eating disorder inexplicably disappeared for five years. At the end of 2009, during Bob's final seven months, I no longer *used* food to navigate life. I was living my days no longer obsessed about food, and my existence was so much richer without the draw of time and energy involved in managing life with an addiction. Who and what I had become without my eating disorder was a revelation to me. I very much admired and respected the woman who emerged. While the event that elicited my first binge after five years of rational eating might have been understandable, I was deeply distraught that I could get caught up in the addiction again. And I did, although to a lesser degree, for another three years. Only recently have I come to understand how and why this happened. Rereading my journal helped.

Wanting to recall these past years accurately, I went back through the journals I had kept intermittently for decades. Throughout my journals, I referenced my distress after a binge, detailing what amounted to a rampage, and then always, I would berate myself and question my character. I would always attempt to unravel why it happened, recounting what I was feeling and what circumstances surrounded the binge. As I read these accounts, it became clear that a binge was unpredictable and was not necessarily related to any circumstance at all. Happy or sad, delighted or annoyed, engaged in a project or bored, I realized that the binges were not simply my way of dealing with old negative tapes running in my head. My belief, reinforced by therapists throughout my many years of disordered eating, was that a binge was circumstantial, that it was fueled by discordance in my life. In other words, I believed that the situations that had formed my childhood and later years contributed to my eating disorder. Therefore, the trigger was my self-perception, accompanied by the demons that unfavorable events or emotions would awaken. This was my belief.

But to the contrary, it was clear that during Bob's illness and impending demise, when circumstances were such that my need to use food for comfort should have been the greatest, I was able to defer to other resources to cope. How did this happen? I will speak later about my final tool of recovery, the purposeful one, the one that I now activate at will. However, back then, the recovery during those five years was unintentional.

A recent consultation with a well-respected evolutionary psychologist, Dr. Jen Howk, helped me understand how, nearly effortlessly, I could bypass this lifelong behavior. Dr. Howk suggested that through these years, my body had become conditioned to the stimulus created by the binge-purge cycle. My "lower brain," the primitive part that considers only basic survival, acclimated to this repetitious response that had become ingrained as a way of dealing with all manner of things in my life. It was a technique perceived as necessary for comfort and survival. She further explained that all actions of humans are based on a cost/benefit analysis, and up to that point, the "benefit" I derived from diving into the numbing process of eating myself into oblivion and then ridding myself of the mayhem served a purpose. It was a behavior and default that my brain came to count on as a kind of comfort and stress release, outweighed by all costs.

Bob's crisis and the shock of my pending and undesirable reality were so demanding in scope that it competed, in my lower brain, with the benefits derived by binge eating. My upper brain, the cerebellum, more specifically, the cerebral cortex—the part of my brain that makes rational decisions and enables action—took control, allowing me to throw myself into the task at hand, that is, caring for my dying husband. This acted as a pattern interrupt, which allowed me the time to experience the benefits of choosing other options. This interruption of habitual behavior allowed for the release of the hold that the addiction had on me. Although this sounds too simplistic, especially considering the intensity and repetitive nature of my eating disorder, I can see that this is precisely what happened. Later, I will return to this and explain it in more detail.

Throughout my years of food fears and struggles, I believed that it was my mind that was directing the actions of my body (through my thoughts and emotions). I thought my mind determined my behavior around food. More specifically, I believed that the resulting thoughts and emotions directed the way I used the food to deal with my present circumstances. From my discussion with Dr. Howk, and a later deep-dive into precepts laid out in a book that turned me completely around (more on that later), it became blatantly clear to me that *it is the type and quality of the food we eat that determines the reactions in our body and that then governs the mental patterns that ensue.*

PART 2:
TAKING CONTROL

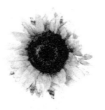

7

THE POWER OF FOOD TO HEAL

In 2018, at sixty-seven, I was growing weary of the physical requirements of my landscape design business. Although a crew of a trusted contractor installed gardens based on my designs, I spent many hours in the sun, overseeing the installations, as well as measuring properties before beginning the design process. It was time for a change, and I began to evaluate my next step: my third career, or as my son, Erik, later coined it, "Mom. 3.0."

Having studied foods and nutrition in college, and being obsessed with the subject from an early age, even while abusing my body when binging, I was drawn to the field of health and nutrition. In the winter of 2017, I enrolled at the Institute of Integrative Nutrition, the largest health coach training institute in the world. After one year of study I became a Certified Integrative Nutrition Health Coach, and I continued my studies by taking their Gut Health course, Hormone Health course, and Health Coach Master class.

While taking these courses, I was exposed to many dietary and lifestyle modalities. Tim and I, both in our late sixties, were open to change, especially because of unfavorable health indicators. Although Tim was the most fearful about the potential regrowth of his pituitary tumor, he was taken aback by blood pressure readings that had become too high. In my case, I blame a one-year experiment with a paleo ketogenic diet for cholesterol that reached over 200, pre-diabetes, and joint pain head-to-foot with high RA antibodies, which indicated that familial rheumatoid arthritis was developing. In addition, gastrointestinal problems were beginning to plague me.

In the conventional medical model, the protocol following unfavorable lab results is to be referred to a specialist, followed by one or more prescriptions for medications to be taken, in many cases, for life. Most medications are not intended to cure but to mitigate symptoms and to bring about better laboratory numbers. Tim and I were not ready to fall into what I felt was the medical black hole. We decided that there would be no medication for us until we allowed Mother Nature to play her hand. Hippocrates said, "Natural forces within us are the true healers of disease." We were ready to listen, and I trusted in the ability of our bodies to heal themselves.

Having read *The Blue Zones,* by Dan Beuttner, about five internationally varied communities with the longest living populations of healthy centenarians in the world, I became convinced that centering our diet on whole plant foods and cutting way back on (or better yet, eliminating) animal products might be the best diet moving forward for us, as it was for all five Blue Zone communities.

In the fall of 2018, I attended a five-day Wellness Forum Health conference in Dayton, Ohio, the focus of which was living healthfully with a plant-based lifestyle. Thus began my indoctrination. After immersing myself in the training and research and enjoying delicious meals prepared with no animal products—no meat, fish, fowl, dairy, cheese, eggs, or butter—I knew I wanted to make the change. Tim, equally as motivated, eagerly followed. By the end of the year, we were both off of all animal products and were reveling in our delicious whole food plant-based meals. We also gave up nearly all processed foods but instead filled our plates with fruits, vegetables, grains, legumes, seeds and nuts, prepared in endless delicious combinations, all bursting with color and flavor. Most important was that, because this is a whole food starch-based nutritional plan, i.e., beans, whole grains (like brown and wild rice, quinoa, oat groats, and buckwheat), sweet and white potatoes, winter squashes, and whole-grain pastas, we felt full and satisfied on these, our comfort foods. Whole food starches are nature's antidepressants. More information on this will follow.

Our choice to shift to a whole food plant-based diet—vegan but without processed plant foods—was validated through our follow-up lab work done in January of 2019, which documented that our health markers were stellar. Our new numbers brought about positive comments from our physicians, but more importantly, we both felt terrific. My joint pain was gone, my cholesterol was down from over 200 to 147, and my blood glucose was in the low 80's, rather than bordering on 120 (which would have indicated diabetes). My gastrointestinal problems were surprisingly mitigated by this fiber-rich diet, although I had been advised to avoid fiber in order to heal my gut. Tim's blood pressure sunk from the 130-140 range to a healthy 110/70 level, where it averages today.

Our greatest concern for Tim came from readings of the MRIs taken during each of his first three years after his 2015 pituitary tumor surgery. The results of each of the three showed a slight amount of tumor regrowth, which concerned the neurosurgeon and prompted him to suggest radiation if, on the follow-up test, the results remained the same. However, after transitioning to a plant-based diet, cutting out all animal products, his two subsequent MRI's (the last in July 2020) showed no additional tumor growth. This may not be conclusive, but it was enough to convince us that we had made the right dietary decision. His neurosurgeon agreed with our conclusion, explaining that he was a lifelong vegetarian.

Dr. T. Collin Campbell, in his highly influential groundbreaking book, *The China Study* (a fundamental book for those considering a whole food plant-based diet for cancer and cardiovascular disease prevention and mitigation), offers strong evidence that animal proteins initiate tissue and tumor growth. Much research has followed, implicating IGF-1 and mTOR pathways in this process. Dr. Campbell's laboratory research proved that he could turn on or off tumor cell growth based on the level of animal protein given. His epidemiological studies involving 6,500 inhabitants in varied Chinese communities produced the same evidence. The research that Dr. Campbell did for this massively wide-ranging study was pivotal in his own decision to adopt a whole food plant-based diet (his terminology) for himself and his family, back in the 1980s, although he came from a multigenerational cattle ranching background.

Based on the work of Dr. Caldwell Esselstyn and his influential book *Prevent and Reverse Heart Disease,* as well as the work of Dr. Alan Goldhamer and his collaborative effort with Dr. Doug Lisle in *The Pleasure Trap,* Tim and I chose to severely limit our intake of sugar, oil, and salt, as well as all processed food. This took some time to implement. But little by little we replaced what came from a factory with what grew in the ground in its most natural state.

Reducing empty calories improved our health noticeably. Choosing to eat food "as grown" greatly removed our temptation to eat "highly palatable food, processed with salt, oil, and sugar in such a way that it hijacks your taste buds" (the subject of *The Pleasure Trap*). This step played an important role in our transition to and love affair with whole, unprocessed food. This also helped us to develop an appreciation for the intricacies of flavors otherwise hidden under a blanket of these dominant and addictive substances.

It is difficult to appreciate the purity and joy of a juicy Honey Crisp apple after eating an apple fritter. Or a buttery, starchy, steamed Yukon Gold potato after eating a bag of greasy, salty potato chips or fries. Simple food like fresh raw vegetables (individually or in huge, delicious salads), bowls of perfectly cooked vegetables, savory black beans, plain brown rice, baked or steamed sweet potatoes, and fresh ripe berries are flavorful beyond belief, but especially once our palettes have adapted to food as it is grown. Trust me, once you transition from processed food (factory manufactured food-like substances) to whole, real food (food as grown), your taste buds will sing and you will be gloriously satisfied.

A surprising side-benefit of transitioning to a whole food plant-based nutritional lifestyle was weight loss for both Tim and me. Unexpectedly, and without trying, I went from feast (usually a binge) or famine (restrictive eating patterns) to deep and nurturing satisfaction with every meal. Throughout my binging years, while following popular belief, I shunned as well as feared, carbohydrates and starches, diligently restricting them. It is not a surprise that when binging, it was processed carbohydrates, sugary treats, and crispy and fried foods that I coveted. They were otherwise forbidden and highly addictive as they took over my brain chemistry, especially dopamine, making me want more and more while finding it hard to stop.

I discovered that starch from healthy whole plant foods calmed me, thereby stabilizing my mood and blood sugar, as well as reducing cravings. This allowed me to feel pleasantly full and completely satisfied after a meal and between meals. For the first time as an adult, I can now eat without counting calories, weighing or measuring portions, or otherwise restricting my food. While enjoying nourishing whole (as opposed to processed) plant-based food, with little to no oil, salt, and sugar, my weight has settled naturally to a new, healthy low of 114 pounds. I gratefully don't feel compelled to obsess about it, or food, any longer. Tim and I love the food that loves us back. This is after a lifetime of weighing myself, sometimes 2-3 times in a day, for most of my adult life. Again, I'm full of gratitude.

Before my full recovery, eating a whole food plant-based diet led to a dramatic reduction in the instances of binge eating. When I fell into the cycle of overeating, then binging and purging, it was more from habit than psychological necessity. It became clear to me that more often than not, I was simply responding to cues, i.e., the urge to do what I had always done when my eating got sloppy and I got too full, or when I was bored, or perhaps otherwise unhappy. It was simply habit, not necessity. The food that was now nourishing me helped me settle into a calmer and more stable place physically, emotionally, and mentally.

It is estimated that 70% of our neurotransmitters are created in our gut microbiome (more on this in "The Power of Food" chapter). It was my experience that the highly nutritious makeup of a whole food plant-based diet and the elimination of processed foods helped to reset my body and mind.

I realized that not only is a whole food plant-based diet the best for health, disease prevention, and longevity (not to mention for animals and the environment), but in my case, it became the cornerstone of my recovery from more than fifty years of addictive, obsessive, compulsive, and erratic behavior related to food. My addiction over the decades is a shame—such a waste in so many ways. I made the best of my life in the areas over which I maintained control, although I mourn that I hadn't found help sooner and regret the decades that I spent living in fear around food. I am grateful, however, for the freedom and sanity of recovery when I finally found it.

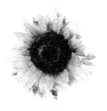

8

THE POWER OF OUR MINDS

Before I take you more deeply into what affected my recovery, I want to emphasize that what I am sharing is based on my personal, individual story. It is impossible to predict or determine the outcome for anyone else who chooses a similar or the same path. In no way do I hold myself out as a recovery expert. The technique described here, and to which I credit my recovery, has had positive effects for many, but sadly not for all.

I also acknowledge those who say that one never really *recovers* from an addiction and others who adamantly deny the existence of food addiction. Some say that by modifying our behavior, we simply hold the addictive behavior at bay. However, until proven differently, the two influencers about whom I am writing strongly believe that the term "recovery" is relevant here, as do I.

It's All in Your Mind

While the first influence I credit in my recovery is my adoption of a highly nourishing, and system-stabilizing, whole food plant-based diet, the second is *Brain Over Binge,* by Kathryn Hansen. Kathryn wrote this honest and heartfelt book in 2011 about her own recovery from disordered eating. In her book, Kathryn explains how she was caught in a vicious cycle of binging and purging (in her case, excessive and punishing exercise) for many years, experiencing no recovery in traditional therapy.

Her breakthrough came after she read *Rational Recovery, The New Cure for Substance Addiction,* by Jack Trimpey, a clinical social worker who made a major breakthrough in the field of addiction to drug, alcohol and substance abuse.

Having read *Rational Recovery,* Kathryn surmised that Mr. Trimpey's Addictive Voice Recognition Technique, or AVRT, might also be applicable to addictive behavior regarding food. She applied his technique, with slight modifications, and very quickly found long-term recovery. During the time that Kathryn was locked in the anguish of her hellish disordered eating, she vowed that if she were ever to recover, she would write a book to help others do the same. I now credit the result of her commitment, *Brain Over Binge,* in part to my own recovery. I also found Jack Trimpey's *Rational Recovery* to be an enlightening and worthwhile read.

After decades of having little to no control over my behavior as it related to food, I overcame the insanity of my lifelong eating disorder within three months with the guidance of *Brain Over Binge* and Hansen's follow up book, *The Brain Over Binge Recovery Guide.* As I write this, I have been free of bulimia for two years, and now, knowing how to activate what I have learned, I cannot ever see myself getting caught in the near death-grip throes of it again.

As it relates to my newfound food freedom, I fully embrace the words of a 1972 song by Johnny Nash:

> *I can see clearly now the rain is gone*
> *I can see all obstacles in my way*
> *Gone are the dark clouds that had me blind*
> *It's gonna be a bright (bright)*
> *Bright (bright) sunshiny day*

I think I can make it now the pain is gone
All of the bad feelings have disappeared
Here is that rainbow I've been praying for
It's gonna be a bright (bright)
Bright (bright) sunshiny day

The Book, The Background, and The Basics

Brain Over Binge led me to the resolution that I was seeking for over fifty years. Within two weeks of reading it and fully embracing the message, I was exercising control over the binge urges, and more often than not, I was actually bypassing them—a new and unfathomable experience for me. Three months later, the binging and purging activity (i.e., my disordered eating) was a thing of the past. Since then, I can't say that my eating has always been perfect, especially during the first year. At times of stress, I ate more than I would have otherwise, finishing a meal feeling too full. Or eating too much of something that was especially rich, or perhaps eating it too fast, the travail of a compulsion.

However, the huge difference during these times was that it was a one-and-done occurrence. Now when any of my old triggers are initiated, no downward spiral ensues. No recrimination. No judgement. No full-on binge. And, most notably, never a purge. A simple observation and acknowledgement, a slight shift, or correction. I have concluded that when this type of behavior happens to most people, it is somewhat innocuous. Therefore, I have chosen to look at it through that same nonjudgmental lens. What freedom! Still, I think of my progress as nearly a miracle when compared to decades and decades of the excruciating alternative.

My most earnest advice to anyone struggling with disordered eating, or any obsessive behavior that presently owns you, is to trust that your life, whatever your circumstance, will be immeasurably better when your behavior is no longer controlled by food. Your emotional relationship with food will be much healthier. Leaving behind a soft, well-worn security blanket (which diving into vast amounts of food can emulate during precarious periods), even when it has outworn its usefulness, can be frightening. It can feel as if a good friend is being left behind and that the road ahead is uncertain, frightening, and possibly lonely. However, nothing can compare with the breathtaking freedom gained when you are no longer owned by a compulsion. Not to mention the pride, self-esteem, and health improvements that are realized on a daily basis.

My early years etched grooves into the record of my life, some tunes of which still haunt me. I have chosen new ways to dance to some of those old rhythms, and some I simply erased, having no need for those old negative songs. In other words, I believe that our past plays a role in our present, but much of our response to it is dependent on how we view it and how we choose to proceed. As I said earlier, life experiences may influence our relationship to food—how, what, and when we eat. But they do not have to. We can be free of repetitive and addictive behavior around food regardless of our past or present life or our emotional state. What I have just described played out in my own life after many, many years of trying to figure it out.

The full title of Kathryn's book is *Brain Over Binge: Why I Was Bulimic, Why Conventional Therapy Didn't Work, and How I Recovered for Good*. I will not, or cannot, in this brief description, present the workable solution that I found in this book. But I can offer the basics. Her general premise, as (in part) taken from Jack Trimpey's book, *Rational Recovery*, is given below. However, it is simplified and shortened and therefore not enough for meaningful action.

The focus of Kathryn's book is to stop binge eating, not to address any other underlying problems a person may be having in their life. In other words, a person can quit right away without having to do anything else first. Although at times, some areas of one's life may need to be worked on in order for that person to be ready to fully take on an eating disorder. But that is not often the case. This method will only work if a person is really desirous of giving up binging. As she puts it, "I believe it can be as simple as this: If you want to be free of binge eating, you are *ready* to be free of binge eating."

Kathryn makes the simple statement that recovery from binge eating comes down to two goals:

1. Learning to dismiss urges to binge
2. Learning to eat adequately

How do we "dismiss urges to binge"? The answer is simple: by understanding the brain. Her initial enlightenment to brain function came from Jack Trimpey, who states that addictive behavior is understandable when viewed in light of the brain. His belief is that addiction comes from an older part of the brain in terms of evolutionary history, what he calls the "animal brain." Kathryn refers to it as the "lower brain." It is responsible for maintaining basic biological functions and ensuring our survival. It is the primitive brain region that generates our drives for food, water, sex, oxygen, and other things it senses are necessary for survival. The lower brain, also called the sub-cortex, is automatic, unthinking, and irrational. It is buried in the central region of the brain and surrounded by the wrinkled outer layer, the cerebral cortex.

When a person is addicted, the animal brain falsely believes that the addictive substance is necessary for survival, and therefore, actually drives the addicted person to the substance, as though it is just as vital as water or oxygen. As it relates to food addiction, Kathryn explains that the lower brain believes that binge eating is a necessity. This is especially true if, at some point, someone experiences an excessive restriction of food, as from anorexia or continual stringent dieting. The animal brain expresses itself through what Trimpey termed the Addictive Voice (AV). Trimpey's writing was geared to substance abuse; therefore, food-based references are in brackets. The AV is "any idea, feeling, or behavior that supports [binge eating]." He says that a [bulimic] must be able to recognize their AV and separate themselves from it because the Addictive Voice is not really their voice, but merely the voice of the lower brain.

Trimpey encourages [bulimics] to observe their own thoughts and feelings using a thinking skill he calls AVRT (Addictive Voice Recognition

Technique). The thoughts and feelings that encourage [binge eating] are the AV, and those that support quitting are the true self. They come from the thinking part of the brain, the cerebellum, especially the frontal lobe, where we make plans, activate goals, control our voluntary behavior, and make intelligent decisions.

When a [bulimic] recognizes and understands their AV, and then completely separates themselves from it, recovery becomes effortless. They must separate from it. Trimpey says that realizing that "It" is merely an appetite that originates in the biological, animal side of human nature allows us to acknowledge that "It" is not really you. It does not direct action, nor does it engage in planning. It guides us to survive based on past experiences, be they pleasure or pain."

In *Brain Over Binge,* Kathryn changes Trimpey's terminology to apply to behaviors around food. For example, the AV (Addictive Voice) is simply referred to as "urges." Throughout her text, we are told to simply STOP listening to those urges and see them for what they are: neurological junk from our lower, primitive, brain. Through neuroplasticity (the moldability of the brain), the more an activity is repeated, the more it becomes dominant; conversely, the less something is expressed, the weaker it becomes, eventually disappearing. This is worth reading a second time—it is a pivotal concept.

In its simplest form, this is the message of *Brain Over Binge* that ultimately changed my behavior. By learning to ignore the urges and see them as neurological junk, little by little, they lost their hold on me. In the end, the urges lost their power to make me respond to them in any way, eventually causing them to disappear, or nearly so. Very rarely, in an intense "triggering" situation, an urge may crop up, directing me to quell it with food. If that happens, it is now so unusual that I actually speak back to it, "Really? Are you kidding? Not on your life, or mine, for that matter!" I then ignore it and go about my business. As she promises, the urge always passes.

Kathryn's second directive for recovery from binging is to eat adequately.

Fortunately, that was not a challenge at all for me because it is built into a low-fat whole-food, plant-based (sans processed food) nutritional plan. To maintain one's weight when eating whole, real food, one must eat adequately and in such a way as to feel comfortably full and satiated after every meal. The starch-based nature of the diet helped me get past the initial anxiety I felt when ignoring an inner voice, that of my lower brain, when for so long, it had total control over my behavior. I cannot say often enough how grateful I am to have learned how to ignore the voice that controlled me so completely for so long!

I will repeat what I suggested above: If you, or someone you know, is struggling with an eating disorder or addictive behavior, reading either or both of these books (as I did) may lead to a final and glorious freedom. In any case, please seek help. Don't do as I did and live for far too long under a secretive shroud of shame. Those lost years of freedom from food fears are my greatest regret.

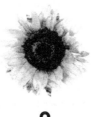

9

AGING WITH POWER

Power, a Noun

Per the Meriam-Webster Dictionary (in bullet-points), power means jurisdiction, control, command, sway, dominion. It implies possession of the ability to wield force, authority, or influence.

To whom but ourselves would we assign power over the process of our aging? And yet, as we age, if we do not implement the strengths defined above as power and do it on our own behalf, who will?

Dylan Thomas, in a cry to his father as he lay dying, wrote

> *Do not go gentle into that good night,*
> *Old age should burn and rave at close of day;*
> *Rage, rage against the dying of the light.*
>
> *Though wise men at their end know dark is right,*
> *Because their words had forked no lightning they*
> *Do not go gentle into that good night.*

The day will certainly come for all of us to go gentle into that good night. Sadly, for some it will be sooner rather than later. For many, certainly sooner than need be. Statistically, more and more of us, at a far younger age than in the past, are becoming burdened with illnesses that are inflicted by poor lifestyle choices, dramatically changing the outcome of our lives. More than two-thirds of all deaths in this country are caused by one or more of these five chronic diseases: heart disease, cancer, stroke, chronic obstructive pulmonary disease and diabetes (An Empirical Study of Chronic Diseases in the United States, March 1, 2018, www.ncbi.nim.nih.gov.pmc). In most cases, these five diseases are related to lifestyle, and it has been clinically proven that a lifestyle medical intervention can often prevent, treat, or even reverse them. More on this in the next chapter.

What is life without good health? The better our health, the richer and more gratifying our lives. The rate of chronic disease in America is climbing precipitously. Disturbingly, that is the case in countries around the world that have been influenced by our unhealthy western diet. It is the dietary standard that has become coined, by many, as the SAD Diet-the Standard American Diet. In other words, we can exercise power—authority, jurisdiction, control, command, sway, and dominion—over how we choose to live our lives, and therefore, over our aging process. To further strengthen and define power, we are in possession of the ability to wield force, authority and influence over our outcome, and, thus, over our lives as we age. And age we will. What is most relevant here is that the level of physical, mental, and emotional health we experience as the years go by is to a great degree under our control and dependent on the lifestyle we choose to live.

As I wrote earlier, our standard of care has become one of ten-to-fifteen-minute conversations with a medical professional, often resulting in a prescription for medication to mediate symptoms—a quick fix, and/or the implementation of a procedure. To be clear, if I break a bone or become ill with a virulent virus (I am writing this at the height of the 2020 COVID-19 pandemic), I will certainly seek conventional medical attention posthaste. However, due to this virus, we have learned more dramatically than ever, (and in many cases, tragically) that the healthier we are and the better that our bodies have been cared for, the greater our chance to avoid illness in the first place and the more rapid our recovery if we do get sick.

A Time to Choose

In the fall of 2018, before my change in diet, my health began to deteriorate dramatically. I was battling two autoimmune diseases, with a third one threatening to damage my joints, potentially crippling me. My physician, and every specialist I consulted, was eager to prescribe medications, all of which were foreign to my body (and hence did not belong there) and would have come with an endless list of side effects. Every new medication would have caused damage in other ways, some requiring further medication to mitigate the effects.

One of the autoimmune diseases was gastrointestinal, and yet, at no time did the gastroenterologist, or any other physician, question what I ate, nor inquire or advise anything regarding my personal lifestyle. Instead, I was prescribed a medication, a biological, that cost my insurance company $1,000 per month, with a personal copay of $225. Food (the right kind) and lifestyle changes, not medication, ultimately resolved all of these autoimmune symptoms.

It was precisely at that time that it became crystal clear to me that my health was heading in the wrong direction. I felt that I had come to a proverbial fork in the road. One path would lead to a lifelong struggle, involving deteriorating health as the years painfully slipped by. The other one would require that I would, without further hesitation, exert personal power over my own health to bring about long-term wellness. Nearly 2,300 years ago, Hippocrates, considered the father of modern medicine, encouraged a vegan dietary protocol and wisely said, "Let food be thy medicine and medicine be thy food." He also advised that "all disease begins in the gut." His overriding belief was that our bodies would heal themselves when given what they need.

Arduous research, fiery determination, and the willingness to make some drastic (and at times, difficult) lifestyle changes led to results that have inspired me to believe that, to a degree, I have aged backwards. No longer feeling arthritic pain nor experiencing stiffness, I can easily squat to recover a dropped pencil without groaning. Having overcome years of gastrointestinal challenges, I can now robustly eat large quantities of high fiber whole food, plates of fruits, vegetables, legumes and starches, without suffering the consequences. Burning with a level of energy that I haven't experienced in many years, I am reveling in taking on new challenges (such as writing this book mere months before my 70th birthday). And my health markers rival that of a person much younger. I am excited about the future!

Gaining Clarity

It was in July 2020 when I grasped the jarring reality that I would be *seventy years old* within six months! It rattled me because it is generally accepted that seventy is "old age." And yet, fifteen months into having made dramatic lifestyle changes, I was feeling better than I had in decades. I'm fit, active, healthy, clear-minded, positive, energetic, grateful, and excited about life.

With those thoughts uppermost in my mind, I began to think about how I wanted to celebrate my seventieth birthday on January 9, 2021. The thought "seventy and soaring" came to mind.

Then another thought occurred to me, inspired by the Blue Zone centenarians: young in mind and body—one-hundred-years old. I allowed myself to think of the beginning of my seventieth year as a great time to launch the *next twenty to thirty years of my life*. Why not? With excitement and expectations of good health and personal growth, why not see into the future with the enthusiasm that I would have if was in my 30s, 40s, or 50s. Although making wise health choices does not guarantee perfect outcomes, the chances of fulfilling my vision of a long and productive life are far greater if the desire and belief are firmly seated in my mind and my heart. May I suggest that you consider doing the same?

I have chosen to embrace what Rhonda Byrne calls "the great mystery of the universe." Her documentary and book, both entitled *The Secret*, ignited a global movement inspired by the premise that personal outcomes and achievements are based on the *law of attraction,* which brings into play all we need when we set our heart, mind, and intention firmly and with conviction on a plan or purpose.

Having read this little book repeatedly, I have seen this law exhibited in my own life, and I now believe that it will again manifest in my life as I enter my third act. If I play my cards right, and my higher power is willing, these upcoming twenty to thirty years are a second chance for me to experience life to a degree that I couldn't when under the cloud of an addictive behavior. I am free to be me, that is, a self-contained, mentally and emotionally stable and mature woman, free from the encumbrance of food fears and compulsions.

There was a time when I could not maneuver through my life without the distraction, crutch, and stress relief offered by my eating disorder. That wasn't living. The person I have become can now clearly see where life is taking me and what I have to offer to others. Another twenty to thirty years is like another lifetime, albeit a shorter one, and I am determined to make these years count. What a blessing and joy it will be!

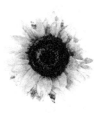

10

THE POWER OF LIFESTYLE

When I gave you the words for this lighthearted song, the anthem of my newfound freedom, I sang them out loud as I wrote them.

I can see clearly now the rain is gone
I can see all obstacles in my way
Gone are the dark clouds that had me blind
It's gonna be a bright shiny day!

These four stanzas apply most directly to the cessation of my eating disorder. However, they also offer clarity as to how I view the direction of my life from here onward, that is, a rebirth, if you will, at seventy years old. I am free of the constrictions from addictive behavior. I am hopeful and enthusiastic about the next 20 to 30 years!

How can I be so brave, or perhaps so brazen, as to put it out there publicly! This confidence in my future has come about from the evidence of the past two years. Both my husband, Tim, and I turned our health around in crucial ways, based on lifestyle decisions and the application thereof. We gained tremendously in health benefits, but more importantly, we are *loving* the positive changes. We are amazed at the healthy and balanced lifestyle we have created. The aged populations in the Blue Zones, those healthy 80, 90, and 100-year-old individuals who inspire us all, have demonstrated that lifestyle decisions have positive effects.

The evidence I see in our personal lives and that of the patients I work with has given me the chutzpah (the great Yiddish word for audacity) to believe that I have power over my own aging process and that I can help others do the same. I needn't elaborate any further than describe these as simple (although not always easy) lifestyle recommendations. In the following chapters, I will offer insight through the acronym, P.O.W.E.R.F.U.L.L.Y., encouraging you to apply these evidence-based lifestyle enhancements to your own life and showing you how.

What is Lifestyle Medicine

In a recent podcast, a physician excused his regrettable lack of information relating to lifestyle as medicine by repeating the admonitions given to him by several of his medical school attending physicians. "Patients don't change. Don't waste your valuable few minutes on counseling; better to use medications, which we know work."

While conducting patient visits, the billable time allotted to physicians is generally dictated by insurance companies and has become greatly restricted. Physicians may offer advice such as "lose weight," "eat a healthy diet," and "exercise more." However, in most conventional-medical practices, there is neither the time nor the protocol for the evaluation of a patient's lifestyle. Yet, a collaborative effort is of paramount importance to get a patient to buy-in and improve outcomes. In this way, lifestyle medicine, the medical model of patient treatment with which I am involved as an Integrative Nutrition Health Coach, shines.

I will offer you a brief history of lifestyle medicine in the U.S. While the specialty of preventive medicine is well known to physicians, lifestyle medicine may be elusive to many. Lifestyle medicine was defined by the Journal of the American Medical Association in 2010 as follows: "The systematic practice of assisting individuals and families to adopt and sustain behaviors that can improve health and quality of life." It embraces the power of simple lifestyle changes to prevent and reverse the progression of the most common chronic diseases, often without drugs or surgery, and without typical side effects other than feeling better.

The American College of Lifestyle Medicine (ACLM), founded in 2004, is a medical professional society of physicians and other professionals dedicated to the clinical and worksite practice of Lifestyle Medicine as their foundation. The practice involves using evidence-based therapeutic approaches such as eating a predominantly whole-food plant-based diet, engaging in age-appropriate regular physical activity, getting adequate sleep, developing stress management practices, being engaged in a caring community, and avoiding the use of risky substances. Added to these positive directives is pursuing other non-drug modalities to treat, reverse, and prevent chronic disease.

Dr. Wayne Dysinger, MD, MPH, is the attending physician and CEO of Lifestyle Medical Riverside, (LifestyleMedical.com), with clinics in Riverside and Redlands, California. I am proud to be affiliated with his successful and growing practice as a health and lifestyle coach. My position involves working with patients individually and in groups, assisting them to clarify and implement the pillars of lifestyle medicine, as well as teaching a monthly whole food plant-based cooking class via Zoom. Dr. Dysinger has historically focused on simply preventing rather than treating disease. He served 12 years as the chairman of the Preventive Medicine Department at his alma mater, the prestigious Loma Linda University, and he is one of the founders of the American College of Lifestyle Medicine, serving as their third president. He is dedicated to broadening the reach of lifestyle medicine nationally, as well as internationally. What good fortune for me that I have the opportunity to practice with a trailblazer of this medical movement that is seeing a doubling every year of physicians becoming Lifestyle Medicine Board-certified.

Passing It On

During my time at Lifestyle Medical, working with Dr. Dysinger and Dr. Pandit, a partnering physician, I have seen scores of patients who start out with multiple chronic diseases, some of which were nearly crippling. They ended up recovering to the degree that they could discontinue all prior medications and could find joy indulging in a vibrantly active lifestyle. Due to this influence, lifestyle remediation and enhancement have become my passion. I apply the fundamentals in my own life and enjoy the benefits daily. I have witnessed that even subtle lifestyle shifts can bring about noteworthy changes in our physical, emotional, and mental wellbeing.

Southern California-based Chef AJ is one of the most admired and outspoken proponents of a vegan diet, and she has recently advised her vast social media audience to find a lifestyle medical physician in order to gain the benefit of the whole-patient care that is offered. On a recent podcast, she was proud to claim that her new lifestyle medical physician is Dr. Dysinger. (You will find hundreds of her insightful interviews and informative cooking classes on YouTube and other platforms—see more about chef AJ's books in "references.")

Aging Powerfully, the title of this book, is a battle cry for meaningful lifestyle changes that we can all adopt, regardless of age. Living long and strong is within the grasp of anyone willing to accept their past, move beyond it, and take control of their future, as I did. Vibrant health, balance, and joy are within reach for anyone willing to engage in the meaningful, evidence-based lifestyle recommendations I outline. Although these pillars of a healthy lifestyle may be simple, change can be hard and can initially appear complex. Consider this book as a straightforward and elementary guidebook for the fundamentals. Throughout, I offer references for further study and direction.

While I learned and grew with the principles of lifestyle as medicine, I read dozens of books, as well as listened to or watched hundreds of podcasts and videos. If you Google any prominent influencer with the word "video" following their name, you can acquire untold hours of free training on any subject. During my daily one- to two-hour morning walk or bike ride, I listen to podcasts. If I find value in the message of the speaker, I will often purchase their book for further research. You will find a list of my favorites in the back of the book. This practice is not only educational but also a very positive method to remain mindful of goals and aspirations as you grow and instill new behaviors into your life.

At the top of my list of lifestyle enhancement resources is *UnDo It!*, written by Dr. Dean Ornish, also a co-founder of the College of Lifestyle Medicine. This New York Times bestseller is a valuable resource for those wanting to fully embrace and apply the fundamentals of evidence-based, results-oriented lifestyle modifications. In *UnDo It!*, Dr. Ornish offers an impressive amount of research, inspiration, and insights on how to make meaningful lifestyle changes. The book is nearly 450 pages long, with more than two hundred pages of recipes and dietary directives, all of which I found invaluable as I was transitioning to a plant-based diet.

(Look for "Dr. Dean and Ann Ornish Want You to Live Better/Rich Roll Podcast" on YouTube or Google, and you can take advantage of Rich Roll's two-hour, highly informative interview of Dr. Ornish and his wife and business partner, Ann.)

PART 3:
AGING P.O.W.E.R.F.U.L.L.Y.

What follows are ten recommendations offered by longevity and lifestyle experts as foundations for vibrant health, calming balance, and meaningful joy. These easily adopted lifestyle fundamentals are among those outlined in *The Blue Zones*. They are also practiced by those who have recovered from terminal cancer, and their stories are told in the remarkable book, *Radical Remission: Surviving Cancer Against All Odds* (more on this to come).

P.O.W.E.R.F.U.L.L.Y consists of two acronyms. P.O.W.E.R. refers to the evidence-based pillars of health as outlined by the College of Lifestyle Medicine, and F.U.L.L.Y. refers to the remaining commonalities of centenarians, as well as terminal patients, who healed themselves.

The pillars of Lifestyle Medicine include Purpose (our why), Others (community), Whole food, plant-heavy (nourishment), Exercise (movement), and Rest (sleep and stress). Although food may be considered the primary determinant of health—after all, we are what we eat—all of these basic principles are vital for overall wellness. Neglect any one of them, and your health may become compromised.

The recommendations represented by the acronym F.U.L.L.Y. are not so much *required* for good, balanced health, but they are insightful additions to bring about wholeness in vibrant health through one's lifestyle. We can, and should, set our sights on aging with *power*—remaining aware and repeating to ourselves often that, in most cases, we do have the *power* to create our own future. We can choose to take our *power* back and wield it to design the life we desire.

As our years go by and signs of advancing age become more evident, many of us relinquish our power and allow fear, uncertainty, and pessimism to set it. Some believe that what is, will remain, that what we have practiced in terms of self-care (or abuse) is too ingrained to change. I also believed that at one time, but now I know that we can redirect our lives at any age.

Many, unfortunately, fall prey to a medical system that, upon recognizing signs of disease, relies on treatment with drugs and procedures rather than promoting lifestyle change for prevention, healing, and, in many cases, reversal. We need to take back our power as patients when we fall into that trap. We must begin, as in the lifestyle as medicine model, with the basic pillars of self-care. With direction and dedication to the principles that I outline below, you can indeed maintain (or reclaim) your *power*.

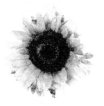

11

THE P.O.W.E.R. OF PURPOSE

Dream in colours, for hues are vibrant.
Paint each day with a smile.
In days of past, don't grieve.
Make new deposits to the pleasant memory bank!
Let your life be a reason for others to LIVE.

~ Somya Kedia

Dan Buettner wrote in *The Blue Zones*, "Okinawans (in Japan) call it *ikigai*, and Nicoyans (in Costa Rica) call it *plan de vida,* but in both cultures the phrase essentially translates to 'why I wake up in the morning.'" He went on to describe an eleven-year-old study funded by the National Institute of Health that looked at the correlation between having a sense of purpose and longevity in individuals between the ages of 65 to 92. The conclusion was that individuals who expressed a clear goal in life—something to get up for in the morning, something that made a difference—lived longer and were sharper than those who did not.

Purpose can arise from something as simple as watching one's children and grandchildren grow up well. It can be a job or a hobby that inspires passion. A new activity such as learning a foreign language or becoming passionate about a cause can ignite an internal fire. In her New York Times bestselling book, *Radical Remission: Surviving Cancer Against All Odds,* Dr. Kelly Turner, a researcher and psychotherapist who specializes in integrative oncology, wrote about more than a thousand cases of radical remission in cancer patients around the world. Each of them defied a terminal cancer diagnosis with a complete reversal of the disease.

In this highly inspiring and informative book, Dr. Turner identified nine key factors that all who recovered had in common. The five P.O.W.E.R. recommendations for lifestyle enhancement are all represented on her list of factors in cancer recovery. What she found as she conducted her interviews was that the patients did not have an "I don't want to die" attitude, but an "I really want to live!" reason for fighting on. They had a zest for life and were excited about the things that they still wanted to do. In fact, they were determined to remain alive deep down in their core.

We don't have to have a terminal illness to muster our determination to live a long, satisfying, and vibrant life. Knowing what we want from life and why we want it, as well as allocating plenty of time to make it happen, turns out to be one of the key secrets to longevity.

Dr. Kelly offers three simple ways to help you make your life more vibrant and meaningful:

1. Write down how many years you want to live. Research has shown that most people who live to be one hundred years old knew with a deep conviction that they wanted to live to that age. Keep your ideal number in your sights. Remind yourself regularly that everything you do today to keep yourself fit and healthy will help bring this goal to fruition.

2. Write your ideal obituary. Regardless of your current health status, this ideal obituary should include the age you would like to reach, who will ideally survive you (e.g. your children and grandchildren) and what accomplishments you would like to be remembered for. This may be an emotional experience, but it is a powerful way to face the fear of death and also to elicit one's deepest desires.

3. Make a list of your current reasons for living and enjoying life, a nice long list of all the things that currently bring you meaning and joy. Put a star next to anything you would like to increase or have more of in your life. Next, make another list of anything new you would like to add to your life to bring you more creativity, happiness, and meaning. Then make it a goal to start bringing these things into your life on a more frequent basis.

Own Your Vision

Where we put our attention is where we tend to end up. The exercises above will help you define your direction. Reflecting on a vision for your life is powerful. Write stream-of-consciousness affirmations to prompts like, "In ten years I want…," as they relate to your health, fitness, relationships, and emotional state, as well as how you spend your time, finances, and contributions in life. This exercise will help you discover what makes you happy and satisfied. You can take this further by asking yourself, "What am I meant to do? Who am I meant to be? What does the universe have in store for me?" "Why do I care?"

My late husband Bob stepped into my life when I was eighteen—after I had an emotionally tumultuous childhood. He loved me enough to help me learn to love myself. Despite my eating disorder, I found peace with the demons that taunted me with the belief that I was unimportant, would never be good enough, and was ultimately unlovable. When I felt loved enough to share my disorder with my husband, we had our son, and I went on to build a sales business that succeeded mightily because I was focused on helping others find the best in themselves, develop their skills, and gain self-esteem. I felt great satisfaction in giving back what had been given to me.

Later, when I was in my fifties, when we sold our company, I became a certified Master Gardener and then a landscape designer. I spent nearly one hundred hours a year volunteering, for ten years, on the Board of the botanic garden of our local university, teaching classes and working with programs to help people learn to create beauty with nature in their own lives. During that period, I felt driven by this purpose, to give back to others in my community.

Six months before turning 70, having been free of the life-long burden of my disordered eating for more than one-and-a-half years, I feel immensely grateful that through lifestyle changes, I am still healthy, fit and full of energy. I was looking at this milestone of age with enthusiasm and a determination to "soar into my seventies." A new thought filled me with excitement: I could and should construct a plan to enter my seventies with purpose to again help others; this time, to coach and guide them to fight current health trends, and to commit to aging powerfully. Science has proven that treating lifestyle as medicine, and following simple steps, will allow us to go into seventies, eighties, nineties, and beyond in vibrant health, satisfying balance, and deep seated joy. Instead of simply hoping to get through my seventies, I now embrace the coming twenty to thirty years as an opportunity to again give back.

It was during this period that I decided to write this book to share my experience and hopefully help others age powerfully by accepting the past and taking control of the future. With clarity of purpose I am committed to do all I can to see this intent through. It simply took finding my vision. I encourage you to likewise find yours.

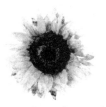

12

THE P.O.W.E.R. OF OTHERS

The best and most beautiful things in the world cannot be seen or even touched - they must be felt with the heart.

~ Helen Keller

If you want to go quickly, go alone.
If you want to go far, go together.

~ African Proverb

In the Lifestyle Medical vernacular, *community* is the term used for our involvement with those around us. Dr. Ornish calls this lifestyle pillar "love more." Dan Buettner, defines this as "the right tribe," explaining that social connectedness is ingrained in the world's Blue Zones. We can also call this concept social support, outreach, and social and spiritual belonging.

In his book, Mr. Buettner explains that Professor Lisa Berkman of Harvard University, who has researched social connectedness and longevity, found that those with the most social connectedness live longer. Of the seniors studied over a nine-year period, those with the least social connectedness were between two to three times more likely to die during the period of the study than those with the most social connectedness. The type of social connectedness was not important in relation to longevity, as long as there was connection. Even the lack of a spouse or significant other could be compensated for by other forms of connection.

Dr. Dean Ornish, in *UnDo It!* writes that the need for authentic connection and community is primal and as fundamental to our health and well-being as the need for air, water, and food. He further explains that loneliness causes chronic emotional stress and overactivation of the sympathetic nervous system. Inflammation increases in people who are lonely or depressed, whereas social support and interaction actually buffers the stress response.

Dr. Ornish defines intimacy as anything that brings us closer together and away from isolation and loneliness. He argues that intimacy is healing. It can be the romantic love of a lover or the platonic intimacy of a friend, child, parent, sibling, teacher, or even a pet. In the case of pets, additional comfort is provided by the unconditional love they offer.

In *Radical Remission,* Dr. Turner reiterates that humans need each other to survive. When surrounded by loved ones, caring acquaintances, or even our pets, the feeling of being cared for releases a flood of potent hormones into our bloodstreams, which not only make us feel better emotionally, but they also strengthen our immune systems significantly. This is one of many reasons that "social support" is one of the key factors in healing for the cancer survivors she wrote about. She estimated that strong social connections were shown to significantly lengthen survival time in critically ill patients by an average of 25%. Dr. Turner stated:

> "What researchers have found through brain MRIs, blood tests, and saliva analysis is that receiving love and social support leads to significant increases in powerful healing hormones such as dopamine, oxytocin serotonin, and endorphins. These hormones in turn boost the immune system by sending signals to decrease inflammation, increase blood and oxygen circulation, and increase the number of white blood cells, red blood cells, helper T cells, and natural killer cells. All these changes help your body

find and remove cancer cells."

Reiterating what we have seen in research, and anecdotally, receiving love from others helps our bodies to remain well. It can be favorable during the treatment of an illness, and it can play a part in the reversal of an otherwise terminal illness.

With the advent of social media and the time invested in this form of socialization, many people have pulled away from more conventional modes of communication. Facebook, for example, might have billions of users, but unfortunately it doesn't really meet the need for authentic intimacy. Most people portray only the best parts of their lives. If we do not bear this in mind, it may appear that everyone else has more confidence, fun, people, and things in their lives, thereby making us feel that we do not measure up. This self-critical thought process further isolates us and is negatively associated with well-being.

At the lifestyle medical family practice I work with, I have conducted nearly two hundred group sessions (many via Zoom during the 2020 COVID-19 pandemic), during which patients have shared their successes and struggles related to their health. They use the pillars of lifestyle medicine as a format that allows for a wide scope of conversation. Patients are open and sincere, receiving acknowledgment and encouragement from fellow attendees. Again and again, they have openly credited these gatherings as an important part of their community and in some cases, their only community, especially in the lock-down phase of the Covid-19 pandemic.

Forgiveness

Estrangement is a negative factor in social connectedness. We cannot consider the importance of community without addressing the subject of forgiveness. The closeness of one person to another, a group, or an organization can be shattered by an inconsequential utterance, a misstep or an action, leading to the long-term destruction of the relationship. The dissolution of the relationship can be detrimental to both parties. I recently came across this truism: even if you are not the violent type, the grudge you might be bitterly holding onto still has the potential to kill, and you are the potential victim.

Anger, resentment, bitterness, and righteous indignation, even when warranted, can have a negative effect on us emotionally, physically, and mentally. Research has shown that a healthy outlook tends to result in greater physical health, while an unhealthy outlook is linked to chronic illness and premature death.

We feel negative emotions four to ten times more intensely than we experience positive ones. At times we revel in events or situations that cause us pain, and they ultimately impair our ability to think and process events. This quote from the Lifestyle Medical Institute CHIP program says it all: "Unforgiveness is like carrying around a red-hot rock with the intention of throwing it at the person who caused you to hurt. But as you wait, the sizzling rock burns and scars your hand. Wouldn't it be wiser just to let the rock fall to the ground? Forgiveness is the skill of letting go."

Do we want our lives to be controlled by another person or an event that took place in the past? Why not set yourself free? An alternative is to forgive and let go of the painful experience and move on, to put the previous incident behind us instead of dragging around the negative memories. One way of letting go is to choose to remember the painful event in a different way. In other words, instead of forgetting what happened, reframe the event. This process requires that we view the situation from another perspective. Is it possible that opposing sides could have behaved differently? This process takes time and is not always easy; however, the alternative may ultimately be far more painful. The rebuilding of previously lost relationships can be tremendously enriching and, back to the point, a valuable move toward building overall health.

Making Connections

Having social connections fulfills an ancestral need to have a tribe. With the knowledge that our health depends upon our interactions, we should consider actions that can be taken to build social connections. Using examples from *The Blue Zones*, Dan Buettner suggests tips for building your inner circle:

Identify Your Inner Circle:
Know the people who reinforce the right habits, those who understand or live by Blue Zone secrets. Go through your address book or contact list of friends. Think about which ones support your healthy habits and challenge you mentally, and which ones you can truly rely on in case of need. Put a big "BZ" by their names. Ideally, family members are the first names on that list.

Be Likable:
Of the centenarians interviewed, there wasn't a grump in the bunch. Dr. Nobuyoshi Hirose, one of Japan's preeminent longevity experts, had a similar observation. Some people are born popular, and people are naturally drawn to them. Likable old people are more apt to have a social network, frequent visitors, and de facto caregivers. They seem to experience less stress and live purposeful lives.

Create Time Together:
Spend at least 30 minutes a day with members of your inner circle. Establish a regular time to meet or share a meal. Take a daily walk. Building a strong friendship requires some effort, but it is an investment that can pay back handsomely in added years.

As I wrote Dan Buettner's recommendations, I couldn't help but ruminate on the current social restrictions that have been levied due to the COVID-19 pandemic. Social distancing. Covering our mouths, and, therefore, our smiles. Think of the closures of many of the venues we typically meet and congregate with new and familiar people. The restaurant down the street with the waitress who, with a knowing smile, simply asks, "your usual?" Or the person at the gym who acknowledges that you are getting stronger. Or, especially, the people at church who greet us with a hug and a blessing.

On the other hand, I have also considered what has become a silver lining in this situation. We have all learned that we can create and be a part of a community virtually. Through Instagram, Facebook, and YouTube, as well as other platforms, we have seen that businesses, and therefore communities, can emerge from the simple act of sharing a positive daily thought, a cooking lesson, or some form of entertainment.

Using Zoom and other meeting apps, we can still gather in groups, and share our thoughts and feelings, while still being heard. In many cases, we can still help families and friends who are separated by distance. We can gather together in multiple locations on a regular basis. In this way, at this time, our electronic devices have advanced our social support systems.

5 Actions to Add Positive Moments to Daily Life
(Psychology Today, July 9, 2019)

1. Even fleeting moments of connection can nourish us. Take a moment to say hello to people as you go through your day: "Hello, how are you!" Then listen to their response. You will find that by doing this during your daily walk or varied activities that you repeat often, it will help you establish valuable connections.

2. Increase your opportunities to interact with others. Join a spiritual group, try an activity at the community center, take a class, or go for a walk in the mall, your neighborhood, or around your office.

3. Engage your strength of kindness and get involved in something larger than yourself. Work at a food pantry, visit a friend or acquaintance who is lonely or ill, offer to help someone by bringing their groceries to their

car. Give up a seat in a waiting area, or let someone get in line in front of you.

4. Share your wellspring of experience. Consider what you may have to offer others—a skill or talent, a helping hand, an impromptu phone call, an invite to lunch—and share from your heart.

5. Reflect on phrases of loving-kindness. This type of compassionate meditation practice evolved from Buddhist origins and can help us open our hearts and feel more interconnected; it can create habits of goodwill toward others (Fredrickson, 2013). In quiet moments of reflection, you might reflect on loving-kindness phrases by directing them toward a particular person or the world in general. Examples of loving-kindness phrases include, "May you be safe. May you be well. May you be happy" (Salzburg, 2010; Fredrickson, 2013). You can develop loving-kindness into a positive habit.

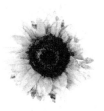

13

THE P.O.<u>W</u>.E.R. OF <u>WHOLE FOODS</u> AND PLANT-STRONG NOURISHMENT

Let food be thy medicine,
and medicine be thy food.

~ Hippocrates

Our bodies are our gardens
to which our wills are gardeners.

~ William Shakespeare

Twenty-three hundred years ago, Hippocrates, the father of modern medicine, himself a vegetarian, advised that a plant-based diet was best for humans, and that the way to good health was through food, primarily plants. He strongly believed that food has the power to adjust, rebalance, and heal our bodies.

More than four hundred years ago, William Shakespeare, also a vegetarian, informed us that we could create the body we desire through our will power—to choose actions that heal and build up our bodies.

The Diet of Blue Zones and "Terminal" Cancer Survivors

Having contracted with National Geographic, and under stringent oversight for accuracy, longevity expert Dan Buettner traveled the globe in search of populations with the oldest citizens who were also happy, healthy, and active. With the assistance of experts from around the world, it took him approximately ten years to identify, verify and document the five areas of the world that he called Blue Zones (having marked in blue potential locations on a map). These areas are Sardinia, Italy; Okinawa, Japan; the Nicoya Peninsula, Costa Rica; Ikaria, Greece; and Loma Linda, California (fifteen minutes from my home).

As he later wrote in the groundbreaking book *The Blue Zones,* all of these populations have a "plant slant" in common. Beans, whole grains, tubers, garden vegetables and fruit, are the cornerstone of their longevity diets, and in some locations, nuts, seeds, and olives are plentiful and enjoyed. Grains are seen as a staple in all Blue Zone diets, as are beans, the primary source of protein. If meat or dairy are eaten, it is in small amounts, in a celebratory way, and, in most cases, not often. The primary longevity diet of the Blue Zones is a whole food plant-strong diet.

In *Radical Remission,* Dr. Kelly Turner, similarly noted that of the more than 1,000 cases she documented of people who recovered from cancer, previously diagnosed as terminal, one of the common healing factors among survivors was their radical change of diet. She noted the four dietary changes made by the majority of them:

- Greatly reduced or eliminated sugar, meat, dairy, and refined foods;

- Greatly increased vegetable and fruit intake;

- Primarily ate organic foods; and

- Primarily drank filtered water.

Those labeled as having had a radical remission from terminal cancer diagnosis (there were stringent requirements used in this evaluation) transitioned to a whole food plant-based diet.

When Dr. T. Colin Campbell coined the phrase "Whole Food Plant-Based (WFPB)" in 1982, he was specifically speaking about whole foods, as close to nature as possible, that are plant-based, or exclusive. Although this is a vegan diet, the term vegan has further implications that he did not want to confuse with his core message. During these past thirty years, after sufficient scientific data accumulation, Dr. Campbell's WFPB guidelines are being adopted by major healthcare and governmental organizations around the world.

Among the organizations that advocate whole food plant-based diets is the Academy of Nutritionists and Dietitians, the American College of Lifestyle Medicine, Medicare: Ornish Reversal Program, Whole Foods: Engine 2 Diet, Kaiser Permanente, the American Association of Clinical Endocrinologists, the American Diabetes Association, the American Medical Association, the American Cancer Society, the World Health Organization, and, in 2020, the United States Department of Agriculture (USDA). (For more on this, see https://gurmeet.ned/food/which organizations-advocate-whole-food-plant-based-diet/index.html).

My dietary preference is a vegan diet (having eaten this way since 2018). However, I consistently use the term "whole food plant-based." The terms "plant-based" and "vegan" refer to a plant-based diet, but they do not necessarily imply healthy food, nor do they guarantee a healthy body. Much of today's junk food is, in fact, vegan. In order to cater to growing consumer demand, food manufacturers are flooding the market with foods labeled "healthy," and yet most of what is being offered is highly processed, with unhealthy levels of oils, refined sugars and salt. Food manufacturers combine oil, sugar, and salt (a combination that you will not find together in nature) in vegan, as well as in conventional foods, in such a way that the resulting processed foods are so highly palatable that they lead to overconsumption.

The more processed food one eats, the less appeal healthy natural foods have. In other words, one becomes trapped in a cycle of overconsumption of artificial, processed, and highly palatable food. *The Pleasure Trap: Mastering the Hidden Force that Undermines Health and Happiness,* by D Lisle, PhD., and A. Goldhamer, CD, explains how we can easily get caught in this phenomenon and what it takes to break free. There are many videos on YouTube in which both doctors independently discuss what they coined "the pleasure trap." Becoming familiar with this concept is very helpful in breaking free from the hold that processed food has on us—and the American population—as evidenced by the growing incidence of lifestyle-related chronic diseases and the decline in life expectancy.

In his book *Spoon Fed: Why Almost Everything You've Been Told About Food Is Wrong,* Tim Spector, PhD. (a professor of Genetic Epidemiology at Kings College, UK), claimed that 50% of the food eaten in England is highly processed; the percentage is even higher at 60% in America. He argues that England has the #1 obesity rate in Europe, and America is #1 in North America. He compared these cases to one of the leanest countries in Europe, Portugal, in which the people consume only 10% of calories from processed food.

Dr. Spector further cited a study in which two groups were given satisfying meals of equal calorie count. One group received meals comprised of whole foods, and the other of highly processed foods. The whole-food group remained full until their next meal. The processed food group became hungry sooner, and therefore they ate more in a day—an average of 30% more calories. The conclusion is that our bodies metabolize processed foods differently than whole foods. Whole, real food is the fuel on which our bodies thrive and maintain high levels of health.

Dr. Spector's book ended with this sentence, "Education is our main hope. We need to be teaching our children about the difference between real and fake food with the same zeal that we teach them to walk, read, and write." He acknowledges that whole food—food that is as close to nature as possible—feeds our microbiome, and therefore, it most perfectly, feeds us.

Processed food, although touted as convenient, healthy, and in some cases, "fuel that our body needs," has been shown to damage our microbiome, and is quite literally killing us.

Why Choose a Whole Food Plant-Based Diet?

Dr. John McDougall wrote in *The Starch Solution* that a whole food plant-based diet is instrumental in preventing "the diseases of affluence." He calls the standard American diet, "the diet of kings and queens." From his observations as a plantation doctor in Hawaii decades ago, those who ate a 60-70% starch-based diet of whole food starches, along with vegetables and fruits, lived long, healthy, and vigorous lives. During subsequent generations, as meat, dairy, and processed foods were added to their diets, their offspring "became fatter, sicker, and died younger." His conclusion, for the past forty years, has been proven: a starch-based, whole food diet will help prevent most chronic diseases.

Another expert who advocates a plant-based diet is Dr. Caldwell Esselstyn Jr., who has documented evidence from 1980 that a whole food plant-based diet, with no oil, salt or sugar, can actually reverse heart disease. He shared the evidence in his ground-breaking book, *Prevent and Reverse Heart Disease,* which also includes recipes that helped me convert to a plant-based diet.

In *Eat to Live,* Dr. Joel Fuhrman emphasizes a "nutritarian diet," which is based on choosing foods specifically for their nutritional excellence. He explains the remarkably beneficial value of phytochemicals and phyto-nutrients, derived from whole food that is plant-based, with an emphasis on those he considers the most valuable nutritionally: G-BOMBS – greens, beans, onions, mushrooms, berries, and seeds (plus nuts).

Dr. Fuhrman sums up a simple concept, "When the ratio of nutrients to calories in the food you eat is high, you lose weight. The more nutrient-dense food you eat, the less you crave fat, sweets, and high calorie foods." Emphasis is put on the variety of nutrients and healing phytochemicals gained from foods specifically based on their color. In other words, a golden beet, and a red beet may both offer nitric oxide, highly desirable for vascular health, but both offer different properties and benefits based on their color. The more colorful the food, the healthier your body is at the cellular level.

Dr. Fuhrman's book is a deep dive into the nutritional value of whole-plant foods and their effect on the body, asserting that this diet will "help you live longer, reduce dependence on medications, and improve your overall health dramatically, and will also change the way you want to eat." Dr. Fuhrman includes a large recipe section in *Eat to Live*, focusing on the most nutritious foods for health—all whole-plant based. Many of these recipes have become staples in my kitchen. You will also find him doing cooking demonstrations on YouTube.

So, What About Our Gut?

Please bear with me as I get a bit nerdy here. In my opinion, the information below ends the debate that some still wage regarding a carbohydrate-heavy, whole food plant-based diet. One of the most relevant concepts to understand about the value of a plant-powered diet relates to our microbiome—those trillions of microbes (bacteria, fungi, viruses, parasites, etc.)—that inhabit not only our guts, but also most surfaces on our body. The microbiome represents a microbial genome that we carry around on and inside ourselves, and that effects nearly every aspect of our health. The results of the ongoing American Gut Project, launched in 2012 from the University of California, San Diego, School of Medicine, were revealed in 2018. The findings about our microbiome (what some simply call our "gut"), and its population of microbes, was revolutionary. As it turns out, our microbiome plays a far greater role in all facets of our health than ever imagined ("First Major Results of 'American Gut Project' Published," May 15, 2018; anesthesiology.duke.edu).

Below are a few observations that were shared so far:

- The number of plant types in a person's diet plays a role in the diversity of their gut microbiome and the number of different types of bacteria living there. No matter the diet they prescribed to (vegan, vegetarian, etc.), participants who ate more than 30 different plant types per week had gut microbiomes that were more diverse than those who ate 10 or fewer.

- Antibiotics affected microbiome diversity; however, those who ate more than 30 plants per week had fewer antibiotic resistant genes in their gut than those who ate 10 or fewer.

- The microbiome of people with mental health disorders, such as depression, schizophrenia, PTSD, and bipolar disorder, tended to be similar to others with the same disorder, rather than with those living in similar situations or with other major factors in common.

According to the findings at the Benoiff Center for Microbiome Medicine at UCSF, published in "Microbiome Perturbation Associates with Disease": "The disturbances of the microbiome can be associated to depression, autism spectrum disorder, oral health, COPD, dermatological problems, cardiovascular disease, asthma, rheumatoid arthritis, IBD, obesity, diabetes, cancer and infection" (The Human Microbiome: A New Frontier in Health; UCTV, December 23, 2019). The health of this three to five pound "organ" (as some call the microbiome), is pivotal to our ongoing health, and fully dependent on what we put into our bodies. "Let food be thy medicine, and medicine be thy food"!

The main metabolites created by the microbiota are short-chain fatty acids (SCFAs) produced in the large intestine through anaerobic fermentation of indigestible polysaccharides, such as dietary fiber and resistant starches (The Role of Short-Chain Fatty Acids from Gut MicrobiotaFrontiers.fendo.2020).

An important part of what makes us healthy are the short chain fatty acids from the plant foods that we eat.

A crucial take away here is that *the only food for the microbiome is fiber*. Only plant foods have fiber! This is crucial, and to a degree, the basis for overall health. It is important to be clear on this important fact. It has become a game for me to count the variety of plant foods that I consume during any given meal, and thus to paint my plate with a gorgeous variety of colors from the foods I have chosen. My husband Tim has gotten into this as well; it is our way of appreciating and celebrating a well-chosen meal.

Although the American Gut Project is ongoing, the study thus far has led to a far greater appreciation for the power of our microbiome to affect our overall health. *Fiber Fueled*, one of the most influential and relevant books specifically about the microbiome, was published in May of 2020 by Dr. Well Bulsiewichz, a board-certified gastroenterologist, internist, and lifestyle medical physician. Dr. B (he encourages this simplified version of his name) has made known that his primary mission in life is to help people find vibrant health by understanding and optimizing their microbiome. And the way that he prescribes that we accomplish this is with the food we eat—a whole food plant-based diet—as part of an overall focus on lifestyle as medicine. He is generously active on social media, where he recently wrote: "Food is the #1 determinant of health and disease in your lifetime. Over the years, you will eat a whopping 80,000 pounds of it. The good news? That means that you get 80,000 chances to make a great choice for your body and your life. Because research shows: Whether it's digestion, metabolism, the immune system, or your mood, all thriving health begins in the gut!" Dr. B's book *Fiber Fueled* is one of the best books on the market about our gut, its effect on our entire body, and most disease systems therein. He has also included a large section of delicious and creative recipes.

There are few in the plant-based world who are more influential than Dr. Michael Greger. On his site, Nutrition Facts.org, he offers a wealth of knowledge on nearly every subject that is health-related. He gives no information that isn't evidence-based. Decades ago he vowed to read every peer-reviewed medical article published, and has generously shared his findings, for free, ever since. He is a treasure trove of credible knowledge, offered in an often-humorous way. He also posts daily, offering very short videos, usually 5-7 minutes and richly informative.

Dr. Greger's best-selling books *How Not to Die* and *How Not to Diet* have become foundational in the plant-based world as he leads us to "Discover the Foods Scientifically Proven to Prevent and Reverse Disease." Dr. Dysinger, the lead physician and founder of Lifestyle Medical, the clinic at which I work, recommends both of these seminal works to his patients. He keeps copies of them in the exam rooms, and he refers often to Dr. Gregor's Daily Dozen foods for health (NutritionFacts.org, Dr. Michael Greger's Daily Dozen).

Tempted to Try a Whole Food Plant-Strong Diet?

In 2018, wanting to improve my health and considering what dietary direction to take, the evidence became so clear to me that the direction became strikingly apparent. The science pointed me to a whole food plant-based diet. Fortunately, with health concerns of his own, my husband Tim was on board. It took us a couple of months to fully transition. Before transitioning, a meal without some form of animal protein seemed incomplete. Now I can't imagine dining on anything other than a variety of radiantly alive, fabulously flavorful, and radically nutritious whole plant-based foods.

In December 2018, I wrote in my journal, "We are now eating four or five meals a week without meat." Several weeks later, I wrote, "We have given up all meat, eggs, milk, and cheese; I can't believe it. We feel great, although I occasionally miss one of my favorites." By January 2019, I wrote with conviction, "We *love* our plant-based meals!" We are capable of neuro-adapting; the longer we avoid a behavior, the less we miss it. The more we repeat a thing, the more that it becomes second nature.

It has been a very long time since we have even considered eating anything but whole-plant foods—legumes, whole grains, vegetables of all kinds, masses of leafy greens, seeds, and nuts. The variety in each of these categories is so great that our meals nearly shout with flavor, not to mention glorious color!

Some people transition to a whole food plant-based diet overnight, which is not uncommon if a life-threatening illness has been diagnosed. However, for some of us it takes a bit of a transition. *The OMD Plan* by Suzy Amis Cameron, may help those who want to ease into a more plant-strong diet. OMD (one meal a day), is Suzy's alternative to a sudden shift by suggesting that one meal a day be fully plant-based. Suzy and James Cameron (producer of *Titanic, Avatar, Terminator,* and many other blockbuster films) both eat exclusively plant-based and are ardent environmentalists. To make her point, Suzy wrote, "Research shows that a plant-based diet is the healthiest on earth; it can help you lose weight, reverse chronic health issues, and improve overall well-being. It's also healthiest for the planet: by swapping meat and dairy for a plant-based meal once a day for a year you can save about 200,000 gallons of water and the carbon equivalent of driving 3,000 miles in your car!" Her book is an inspiring read, and it includes her creative and delicious plant-based recipes.

For a comprehensive look at eating for health as well as for the planet, consider watching *Eating You Alive:* a feature-length documentary revealing the truth behind why Americans are so sick and what we can do about it. James Cameron, Samuel L Jackson, and Suzy Amis Cameron are part of the production team. You can find it on YouTube as well as other platforms. Other inspirational and informative films include, *Forks Over Knives, Cowspiracy, What the Health*, and *The Game Changers*.

I intended this book to be fundamental and foundational, and therefore, not specifically directive. With that being said, I will recommend a little book, *The Vegan Starter Kit,* that will be very instrumental in transitioning to plant-based eating, especially for those who want to ease into it. The best-selling author of more than 13 books, Dr. Neal D. Barnard is perhaps the world's most respected authority on vegan diets. This guide will assist anyone who wants to transition to a plant-based diet. He offers step-by-step suggestions toward adopting a more plant-forward way of eating.

Many people have explained to me that they could not tolerate beans, raw vegetables, grains, or nuts, etc. It is important to understand that our digestive systems, as well as our microbiomes, have been "trained" by what we have habitually fed them. Dr. B., in *Fiber Fueled,* does a very good of explaining this and helping one understand how to retrain our system. The more we eat a diverse whole-plant-food diet, the better that we will tolerate it. Those who continue to eat animal products can still realize a huge boost to their overall health by adding more and more plant-based, unprocessed foods. Our microbiome, and therefore our entire system, including our brain, will thank you for it!

One last thought about this pillar of health that we call "nourishment." While I work with patients toward an optimal diet at Lifestyle Medical, we take a whole-body approach. There is no doubt that what we put in our bodies can heal or harm us, and that what enters our body is more than just the food we eat. It is what we drink, whether or not we smoke, the drugs that we take, the cosmetics and lotions that we apply to our skin, the products we use to clean our homes, electromagnetic radiation, and environmental toxins.

With this in mind, I have not only cleaned up my diet by eating what I consider to be the most nourishing and health-giving food for my body, but I have also cleaned up my environment. To this end, my food is organic, thereby avoiding pesticides and herbicides (especially glyphosate). My drink of choice is filtered water from reverse osmosis tap in my kitchen, poured into stainless steel or glass, not plastic. Commercial drugs and medications of all kinds are avoided when possible. The cosmetics that I buy are "clean" and checked against the Environmental Working Groups lists of commercial toxins. I keep in mind that what enters through the skin enters the bloodstream and can have a greater effect than what enters through the gastrointestinal tract. My household cleaning supplies are free of harsh chemicals and fragrances (see references for a book that helps with this). Breathing fresh air, especially out in nature, positively affects our system and is therefore something that I incorporate into every day.

Although this may be less understood, I am also very mindful of EMF radiation (electromagnetic frequency), which I measure with a meter (see references). I have been amazed by the readings of some of the otherwise innocuous devices. For example, a white noise machine and a baby monitor (for a visiting grandchild) both had surprisingly high readings. Knowing this allowed me to place them at a distance for safety or to discontinue their use, if warranted. For example, when the readings on my twenty-five-year-old built-in oven and dishwasher were nearly off-the-chart while not in use, I replaced them both as soon as possible. In this case, knowledge was power in that until they were removed, I limited the time that I worked near them in the kitchen. There are those who say that electromagnetic radiation is innocuous. There are those who say that it affects us at a cellular level. My feeling is that I will proceed with caution based on the evidence that I have seen.

You Hold the Key

As we age with power and grace, we want to remain mindful that to experience vibrant health, balance, and joy, each of the pillars of lifestyle matters. However, nothing will affect us more directly and dramatically as what we put in, on, and around our bodies.

The Seventh Day Adventists of Loma Linda, California, the only Blue Zone community in America, believe that our body is a temple, a gift from God. Although they are surrounded by intense commercialization as it relates to food, social influences, and environmental pollution, their dietary and lifestyle practices are prescribed by their religious teachings, which has led to the largest group of vegans and pure vegetarians of all the Blue Zones. On average, they live ten healthy, happy, and vigorous years longer than the average American. While living a city life in America, they can lay claim to being one of the longest-lived people in the world. They are aging powerfully. If they can, we all can, one forkful at a time.

I will finish this chapter by saying that simply adding more whole-plant foods to your diet can be a game-changer. The more, the better. Honestly, every whole-plant food that makes it into your gut creates a system-wide positive affect. Listen to your mother, "Eat your vegetables!"

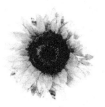

14

THE P.O.W.E.R. OF <u>EXERCISE</u>

When it comes to health and well-being,
regular exercise is about as close
to a magic potion as you can get.

~ Tich Nhat Hanh

The doctor of the future will give no medicine,
but will involve the patient in the proper use of food,
fresh air, and exercise.

~ Thomas Edison

What do a Vietnamese Buddhist monk and the father of invention have in common? Clearly, they know that our bodies are meant to move. We cannot have health nor well-being without exercise, which we define in lifestyle medicine as *movement.*

Dan Buettner shared this about the centenarians featured in *Blue Zones,* "Longevity all-stars don't run marathons or compete in triathlons; they don't transform themselves into weekend warriors on Saturday mornings. Instead, they engage in regular, low-intensity physical activity, often as part of a daily work routine." Movement. Living life on the go. Bypassing conveniences for full involvement.

He went on to explain that the inhabitants of Blue Zones move naturally throughout the day. They garden in Okinawa while growing their own food; hike in Sardinia while shepherding; care for grandchildren and visiting neighbors in hilly Ikaria; and go on nature walks in Loma Linda, California.

In *The Alzheimer's Solution*, doctors Dean and Ayesha Sherzai, both MDs and neurologists, explained that exercise is crucial for long-term brain health. More specifically, they argue that both aerobic and resistance training are remarkably effective at protecting the brain against age-related decline, including the possibility of reversing the symptoms of early Alzheimer's. As codirectors of the *Brain Health and Alzheimer's Prevention Program* at Loma Linda University Medical Center, the Sherzais promote the importance of lifestyle as medicine and emphasize that sedentary behaviors have been associated with many types of chronic disease, including cognitive impairment. In fact, exercise is crucial for every system of the body, especially the brain.

In their excellent book, as much about lifestyle modalities as the specifics of brain health, they address what some have come to consider "normal aging," the limiting beliefs we have set for ourselves with low expectations. They stress that human physiology is capable of remarkable things at age sixty, seventy, eighty and beyond, offering the example of a colleague at Loma Linda University, Dr. Ellsworth Wareham, who participated in open-heart surgeries until he was 95. Drs. Sherzai implore us to challenge our assumptions regarding the physical limitations of mid- and late-life and instead choose to age powerfully (my words) by rejecting our preconceived limitations. They insist that our brains cannot age well if our bodies are not used as designed, that is, to move well and often. In their excellent chapter on exercise, they outline strategies for creating a personalized exercise program. In addition, there are many free and age-appropriate programs to be found online by simply searching Google or YouTube.

Dr. Dean Ornish emphasized that exercise will help you live longer, be happier, and give you a more vibrant life. It will offer a source of recreation, protect you from disease, and make you happier due to the endorphins released by exercise. In *UnDo It!*, his chapter on exercise illustrates valuable resistance training that can be done at home with simple exercise bands, as well as yoga-inspired stretches that will keep every area of the body loose and limber.

Sit Less, Move More

We live in an environment geared toward inactivity, so it is little wonder that our default mode as a society is to be underactive. It has become clear that there are long-term consequences of too much sitting and not enough moving, even among those who have a daily exercise regime but then spend most of the day sitting.

As reported by the Lifestyle Medicine Institute, in a study of more than 120,000 adults monitored for 14 years, people who sat for extended periods in their leisure time and did not exercise had a greatly increased risk of premature death. It showed a 94 percent increase for women and a 48 percent increase for men. The researchers found that those individuals who exercised regularly but then sat for extended periods during the day nevertheless had a greatly increased early death rate. It is conclusive; we are meant to move, and to move regularly.

In their Complete Health Improvement Program, the Lifestyle Medicine Institute offers practical tips for sitting less and moving more:

At Home:
- Move around the house while talking on the phone.
- Stand up and walk around the house during TV commercial breaks.
- Do household chores that involve standing, such as ironing, while watching TV.
- Stand and read the mail, magazine articles, and emails.

At Work:

- Stand and take a break from your computer every 30 minutes.

- Stand periodically during long meetings. When asked about it, explain why. This may encourage others to join you.

- Stand to greet visitors and when taking phone calls.

- Drink more water so that you have to go for refills, and to visit the bathroom: thus, more movement.

- Move items like the trash can, filing cabinet, printer, etc., out of reach to encourage standing.

- Consider a standing desk and encourage "stand while we talk" meetings.

- Stand at the back of the room during presentations.

- Eat your lunch away from your desk, preferably a distance away from the office, and walk there.

- Walk during part of lunch and/or breaks.

When Out and About:

- Park your car a distance from your destination and walk.

- Plan regular breaks during long car rides.

- Use public transportation in order to walk to and from stops or stations.

- Whenever possible, offer your seat to someone who needs it. Enjoy standing.

Purposeful Exercise

Speak to your physician first if you have not enjoyed movement in the past. When you are given the green light, or if you are already comfortable moving, set a goal to move continuously for at least 30 minutes a day and at least three days a week. Build to one hour or more, five to seven days a week if possible.

My recommendations reflect my own lifestyle. Beginning in my early twenties, I built movement into my daily routine. Even at seventy years old, my husband and I roll out of bed early every morning, throw on our work-out clothes, and take off for an hour-long hike on a local mountain trail. Or, we might take a long bike ride on a nearby river-bottom trail, and around a city park with geese in the lake. My treat is the sheer enjoyment of movement, the sights and sounds, as well as the ability to listen while I move to an interesting and relevant podcast.

On the days that we take our mountain trail walk, my husband listens to podcasts with me. This has kept us on the same page with dietary, health, environmental, and social issues. We also end our evenings with a 30-minute after-dinner walk to discuss the day. Again, it's a rewarding experience. This commitment to move has kept my body limber, fit, and comfortable with movement. I fully embrace the adage, "Move it or lose it."

The best exercise program is the one you will actually do! Reward yourself for the movement. Do something that you look forward to, or that you consider a treat. For example, weight loss expert Chef AJ, author of *Unprocessed, The Secrets of Ultimate Weight Loss*, and the *75-recipe section of Own Your Health*, rewards herself during her morning spin-bike session with a Netflix program she is anxious to watch. A couple in their seventies, both patients with whom I work, play an active game of disc golf (free at a local park) a couple of times a week for fun and a thorough workout, and they enjoy cycling. Another patient, who spends most of her days on a mobile scooter, joins a senior center group on Zoom several times a week for chair aerobics, reveling in the camaraderie, the energetic movement, and the satisfaction of accomplishment.

What Counts?

Add more to your everyday movement. Take the stairs whenever possible; try two at a time while you hold on to the rail for balance. Choose a parking spot in the back of the lot and enjoy the walk as well as the relief from congested parking aisles. Clean house to your favorite jazzy music and move to the beat. Fidget more: tap your toes, twitch your legs, make exaggerated arm movements, and/or take laps around the room while you are on the phone.

Take a brisk walk (walking your dog counts here). Ride your bike. Swim. Play tennis or golf. Using bands, weights, or your own body, do resistance training—even if it is as simple as doing proper squats while you squeegee in the shower. Join a yoga group on Zoom or take a class. Consider chair aerobics. Create a garden and care for it regularly. Join a walking group. Enter a walk or run 5K. Visit a local botanic garden. Walk to the store for your favorite piece of fruit or a good cup of coffee. Turn on some lively music and dance till you drop. Play frisbee with whoever will play. Plan a walking meeting with workmates or friends. Take a dance class such as tap, ballet, salsa, or swing, and enjoy your new skills. In the heat of summer, have a water balloon battle. Master a jump rope routine. Pull out your old hula hoop or buy a new one. Join a sports team. Make date-night an active one with miniature golf, laser tag or dancing. Enjoy a trampoline; minis are fun too. Go camping and hike the trails. Even engaging in isometrics counts here. Squeeze those butt cheeks, hold, and relax. Actually, *anything* that you enjoy doing that involves sustained movement counts. Remind yourself to move it, or you will lose it!

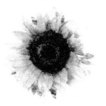

15

THE P.O.W.E.R. OF REST

Verb: Rest. To stop working or moving in order to relax or recover your strength.
Noun: Rest. 1. A period of resting. 2. A motionless state.

Noun: Resilience. Adjective: Resilient. 1. Able to spring back into shape after bending, stretching, or being compressed. 2. Able to withstand or recover quickly from a difficult condition. 3. The ability of a person to adjust to or recover readily from illness, adversity, major life changes, etc.

It is taken for granted by many, including myself, that the most important factor in maintaining health relates to what we put in our bodies. I've always considered nourishment to be the go-to lifestyle fix for whatever ails us. The lifestyle pillar of nourishment, especially nourishment that is whole food plant-based, is one that I have promoted most energetically. The pillar of rest, or as we call it in my Lifestyle Medical office, resilience, encompasses sleep, stress relief, mindfulness, and meditation. It has been taken somewhat for granted by many as a mere recommendation rather than an imperative. As for myself, I had a wake-up call about resilience.

Despite my dietary choices that cover a full spectrum of colors and variety and the powerful nourishment and benefits of whole plant-based meals, my otherwise healthy operating system suddenly developed a snafu. My G.I. tract began to misfire, and things stopped working as well as I had come to expect. Unhappy and puzzled, I began to review what I was eating, evaluating what foods might have "turned on me." Simultaneously I began writing this chapter, and the light went on. It was two weeks before Thanksgiving. I was about to have two rounds of house guests. I had further underestimated the recovery time of a surgery scheduled for the week prior to Thanksgiving. And most disconcerting, the manuscript for this book had been promised to the editor within this time frame.

While writing about the pillars of lifestyle, I had been working into the night, sleeping no more than six hours a night (rather than my preferred seven to eight), worrying about outcomes, and harboring a constant knot in my stomach, neck and shoulders. Oddly, because this is a coveted and meaningful project, I dismissed all the physical ramifications that this continual system-wide disruption might have on me. I didn't even acknowledge the signs when they appeared.

Having a very goal-driven personality, it took me two days to accept the truth after I recognized it, primarily because I have a bring-it-on way of dealing with challenges, and I take pride in handling things coming from all directions.

Resilience. Although I teach about this lifestyle medical pillar of health and the habits that most affect our central nervous system, I had not previously embraced the true consequences of not giving the subject of rest it's just due. This is no longer the case.

Once I recognized what was happening to me (actually, when I began the research for this chapter), I called my book publisher and set a more attainable due date, although still in time for my much-anticipated seventieth birthday and book launch party on January 9, 2021. Immediately, I felt a weight lifted off of my chest, and I could take deep breaths again. Bowing out of hosting my son's family during the Thanksgiving weekend (a painful decision) was smart and necessary, especially one-week post-surgery.

More pressure was relieved, and I felt the knot in my stomach unravel. Reframing my writing time alleviated stress, as did committing to intersperse a walking meditation practice between my daily podcasts, which fire up my brain and excite me with even more must-do ideas. Finally, having foolishly allowed my daily morning and evening meditation practice to get messy and much less focused, I recommitted and became diligent again. What a relief! A heavy self-imposed shroud was lifted, and in less than one week, my system was functioning beautifully again. Resilience. We can eat well, move more, and have great social ties, but if we are sleep deprived and anxious, our bodies will nevertheless rebel. Symptoms of the discordance will then become evident.

The Necessity and Benefits of Sleep

Let's get right to the science. It has been scientifically proven that restorative sleep (or a lack thereof) influences our cognition and our health. In their book, *The Alzheimer's Solution,* doctors Dean and Ayesha Sherzai write that "Sleep was designed especially for the brain. Our bodies are bound by an automatic daily cycle, shifting back and forth between wakefulness and passive rest, but the brain enters a completely different state during sleep. This energetic state promotes two important functions: 1) Detoxification of amyloid and oxidative by-products; and 2) Consolidation of memory and thought: short term memories are converted into long-term memories, unneeded memories are eliminated, thought processes are organized, and new connections built." This being so, it is stunning that as a society, we are so cavalier about our sleep and often, a lack thereof.

The Sherzais offer an outline of thirteen essential health parameters affected by sleep (with references noted in the book):

- **Overall health:** People who sleep better spend less time at the doctor's office. Getting quality sleep reduces your risk for our most common chronic diseases: heart disease, stroke, Alzheimer's, and diabetes.

- **Immunity:** Better sleep leads to fewer colds and immune-related disorders, and even a lower risk of cancer. Restorative sleep has a particularly profound effect on the body's response to inflammation. Lowering inflammation decreases the risk of developing Alzheimer's.

- **Mood:** People who sleep appropriately are happier. There is a direct correlation between restorative sleep and both qualitative and quantitative measures of happiness. Many studies have indicated that quality sleep results in better mood, insight, social engagement, and overall quality of life.

- **Focus and attention:** Focus and attention are the foundation of cognition and complex functions like visuospatial and motor skills. Both are impaired by lack of sleep and improved by proper sleep. Insufficient sleep affects the way we perceive and process information.

- **Learning:** People who sleep well have better short-term and long-term memory, processing speed, recall, visuospatial skills, driving skills, and even athletic skills.

- **Coordination:** A lack of sleep can blunt our responses to the environment, making us more likely to drop objects and struggle with intricate or even simple actions.

- **Decision making:** People who sleep regularly are less likely to make bad financial decisions. Sleep-deprived individuals tend to be biased toward inappropriate risks. It appears that sleeplessness inhibits the frontal lobe, causing you to favor immediate, visceral choices over more complex ones.

- **Alcohol and drug abuse:** Good sleepers are less likely to abuse alcohol and other drugs, again, related to the frontal lobe's ability to inhibit inappropriate choices. Restful sleep makes you much less likely to abuse substances that will negatively affect your cognition.

- **Diabetes:** People who don't sleep enough are more likely to develop type 2 diabetes. Studies have shown a direct link between sleep and the body's ability to process insulin. Adults who sleep seven to eight hours per night (compared to those who get six hours) are 1.7 times less likely to develop diabetes. In fact, those who sleep five hours are 2.3 times more likely to develop diabetes.

- **Stroke:** A lack of quality sleep increases the risk of stroke. Sleep is crucial to healthy vascular function.

- **Headaches:** People who sleep better experience far fewer migraines and tension headaches. After forty-three women were trained to improve their sleep with sleep hygiene techniques, all the participants except one experienced fewer headaches, and most were headache free for long periods.

- **Weight regulation:** In a thirteen-year study of 500 individuals, researchers found that those who regularly sleep less than seven hours per night are 7.5 times more likely to be overweight, even after controlling for activity levels and family history. Reasons for this include the inhibition of the frontal lobe, which leads to the vulnerability of cravings and abnormal circadian rhythms that affect the brain's satiety and hunger centers. Sleep deprivation causes cravings for high-fat foods and sweets, which contribute to spikes in hormones that increase the appetite, thereby leading to more snacking.

- **Libido:** People who get more sleep have a better libido and increased testosterone levels. A low libido can cause depression and a diminished quality of life, both of which affect cognition and memory.

- **Brain atrophy:** Sleep deprivation can cause microglia (the brain's specialized waste clearance cells) to destroy healthy neurons and their connections. This innate detox system is essential for clearing harmful by-products, but when we're chronically sleep-deprived, the system turns on itself, pruning the cells it is meant to preserve. This may explain brain shrinkage in those individuals who are chronically sleep-deprived.

Although the Sherzais are both neurologists who focus on the brain, they are also board certified with the College of Lifestyle Medicine and are keenly aware of all facets of healthy living. Therefore, every aspect of lifestyle as medicine is covered in their excellent book. Regarding sleep, they strongly recommend that we get no fewer than six hours of sleep per night and that we average at least seven to eight hours, although they stress that it's the quality of sleep that matters most. Quality sleep is restorative sleep that leaves you feeling refreshed.

Sleep Hygiene

From the Sherzais outline of health deficits due to a lack of sleep, it is clear that a good night's sleep is crucial. Allowing for individual parameters, this is typically described as seven to eight hours per night. It will vary with clinical disorders such as insomnia, narcolepsy, restless leg syndrome and sleep apnea. Our sleep patterns are something we influence by implementing certain habits, and they are often referred to collectively as *sleep hygiene*.

Note: If you suspect that your inability to sleep has clinical undertones, you will want to receive an evaluation by a healthcare provider.

Our behaviors during the day, especially before bedtime, have an impact on our sleep: promoting healthy sleep or leaving us sleep-deprived. What we eat and drink, the medications we take, how we schedule our days and choose to spend our evenings can significantly alter our quality of sleep. Below you will find a list of healthy sleep habits that you may find will positively impact your quality of sleep.

- Keep a consistent sleep schedule: getting up at the same time every day, even on weekends or during vacations.

- Set a bedtime early enough for you to get at least 7 hours of sleep.

- Establish a relaxing bedtime routine.

- Use your bed only for sleep and sex.

- Make your bedroom quiet and relaxing. Keep the room at a comfortable, cool temperature.

- Limit exposure to bright light in the evenings (especially blue light from electronic devices), and get bright natural light first thing in the morning. Preferably, outdoors in the sun.

- Turn off electronic devices at least 30 minutes before bedtime. Also, avoid playing games and watching stimulating movies.

- Don't eat a large meal before bedtime and avoid eating late at night in general.

- Exercise regularly, but avoid exercising before sleep.

- Avoid consuming caffeine in the late afternoon and evening. If you are overly sensitive to caffeine, avoid it altogether.

- Use meditation as part of your pre-bedtime routine.

- Avoid alcohol before bedtime.

- Reduce fluid intake before bedtime.

- Sound and light-proof your bedroom. Use blackout curtains or shades, and consider white noise or natural soft sounds.

Foods that can be especially disruptive to sleep include:

- Sugary foods that give your body quick energy but that interfere with relaxation and sleep

- High-fat foods that can cause indigestion and acid reflux

- Spicy foods that can irritate the stomach and also cause acid reflux

- Chocolate, which contains sugar and caffeine, both of which affect sleep

Stress, from Inside and Out

You're running late, driving a bit too fast, and worried about what you will miss by being late. Suddenly, in the rear-view mirror, you see a flashing red light. What happens next? The "stress response" kicks in: racing pulse, sweaty palms, tense muscles, unsettled stomach and more. The sympathetic response of your autonomic nervous system has sent you into fight-or-flight mode—an ancient protective mode helpful when the adrenaline is actually needed. Stress is an unavoidable part of living; however, when chronically activated, our health will be adversely affected and our bodies will suffer.

In the last twenty years or so, research has begun to support the theory that letting go of suppressed emotions, pent up anger, and resentment can be beneficial to the physical body. This is especially true of stress. A landmark stress study was published in the New England Journal of Medicine in 1992 ("Psychological Stress and Susceptibility to the Common Cold") in which more than 420 men and women were given surveys on a variety of factors, stress being one of them. They were then exposed to the common cold virus. The results of this study very clearly indicated that of all the factors evaluated, stress was clearly implicated in whether or not the individuals would develop a full-on cold. Since then, hundreds of studies have shown that stress weakens the immune system and is associated not only with the common cold but also with chronic diseases like heart disease, autoimmune disorders, and cancer.

Stress serves an important purpose in that it enables us to respond quickly to threats and avoid danger. However, lengthy exposure to stress may lead to mental health difficulties such as anxiety and depression, or as discussed above, to increased physical health problems.

While we cannot avoid all stress, we can work to handle it in healthy ways that increase our potential to recover:

- Eat and drink to optimize health. Add more antioxidant-rich and nutritionally dense whole-plant foods to your diet. Although people try to reduce stress by drinking alcohol, using tobacco or eating too much, these actions actually add stress in the long run. Caffeine also can compound the effects of stress.

- Exercise regularly. In addition to having physical health benefits, exercise is a powerful stress reliever. Movement activities like yoga and Tai Chi have the additional benefit of focusing on mindfulness and breathing.

- Meditate and practice relaxation techniques. Meditation will instill a sense of calm, peace, and balance that can benefit both your emotional well-being and your overall health. Guided meditation, guided imagery, visualization, and other forms of meditation can be practiced anywhere at any time, whether you are out for a walk, riding the bus to work, or waiting for an appointment. There are many free apps online to get you started. You can also try deep breathing anywhere. Simply take a long deep inhale through your nose and a steady and full exhale through your mouth.

- Don't go it alone. Social contact is a good stress reliever because it offers a distraction, provides support, and helps you navigate life's ups and downs. Make a call, meet a friend for coffee or a meal, email a friend or family member, or visit your place of worship. Opportunities to volunteer can also add richness to your community and give a stress-relieving sense of satisfaction. (Check out volunteermatch. com).

- Reduce stress triggers. If you find that your life is filled with too many demands and too little time, reevaluate what matters, what resonates with you, and how you could better manage your time. You can relieve some of these demands by asking for help when it's appropriate, setting priorities, pacing yourself, and reserving time for self-care.

- Just say "NO" to demands on your time and energy that will place too much stress on you. Do not feel obliged to meet the expectations of others. Assert yourself when necessary.

- Get enough sleep. The quality and amount you get can affect how stressors impact you.

- Keep a journal. Writing down your thoughts and feelings can be a good release for otherwise pent-up emotions. Don't think about what to write. Just let it flow. Write whatever comes to mind. No one else needs to read it, so don't strive for perfection in grammar and spelling.

- Get musical. Listening to or playing music is a good stress reliever because these activities can provide a mental distraction, reduce muscle tension, and decrease stress hormones. If you like, crank up the volume and let your mind become absorbed by the music.

- Seek counseling. If stressors are challenging your ability to cope or if self-care is being neglected, consider asking for help from a professional.

- Practice stress-relieving self-care. Treat yourself to a massage as often as possible. Take Epsom salt baths. Employ an arsenal of calming essential oils in your bath, in a diffuser, on your pillow or on your skin, possibly with a carrier cream. Use them singularly or blended. Some of the best de-stressors include lavender, lemon balm, neroli, ylang-ylang, angelica root, geranium, sage, and grapefruit.

A Few Techniques

Mindfulness is the basic human ability to be fully present and aware of where we are and what we are doing. Mindful breathing can trigger a calming reaction known as the parasympathetic response, or as rest and digest (another branch of the autonomic nervous system) that brings about a feeling of calm and relaxation. Studies have shown that breathwork can change our states of being. There are many forms of mindful breathing. Simply taking several deep breaths through the nose and out through the mouth can help relax you.

Andrew Huberman, PhD. (@hubermanlab) is a neuroscientist and Professor of Neurobiology at Stanford University School of Medicine, and leader of the Huberman Lab. In an effort to educate the masses and share neuroscience in words that are easy to understand, he has taken to social media to share his message on the use of our breath and eyes to control our physiology. In an insightful interview, *How to Change Your Brain* (on YouTube), with Rich Roll (ultra-endurance athlete, vegan dietary advocate, and international speaker), Dr. Huberman shared what his lab claims to be the most effective breathing technique to release stress.

He explained a rather simple method, calling it a *physiological sigh*. To paraphrase him, "Before you begin, take a regular inhalation and exhalation. Then take a sharp, nearly full inhale, with an additional inhale near the top of the first. And then a full release of all of the breath." That's it. I practice this regularly when I catch myself tensing up, and I instantly feel the difference.

Box Breathing (the Navy Seal breathing technique) can be used to calm yourself down. The technique is simple:

1. Inhale for 4 seconds
2. Hold your lungs full for 4 seconds
3. Exhale for 4 seconds
4. Hold your lungs empty for 4 seconds

Walking Meditation is a tool to develop embodied awareness and a way to develop feelings of calm and appreciation for the world around us. It's a way to enter into a state of peace and calm. This can be practiced anywhere, but outside, especially in nature, is best. Walk at a natural, moderate pace and pay attention to the sensations on the bottom of your feet as each foot touches the ground. Then shift your attention to what you see—the colors, shapes, light and shadows. Simply observe. Next, shift attention to what you hear. Distant cars? Birds? Children playing? Dogs barking? No judgement. Just observe. Take your focus back to your footsteps, then back to reality.

Progressive Muscle Relaxation. This practice helps reduce stress and anxiety by tensing the body and then relaxing it. While lying down or sitting, take a few deep breaths, in through the nose, out through the mouth. Then, beginning at your feet, curl your toes and feet with gentle pressure. Hold to a count of five, then relax. This can be a brief or prolonged exercise, depending on the number of body parts that are tensed and then relaxed. I usually chose ten, followed by an overall tensing of the body, and then total relaxation. By practicing this, we become more aware of how both states feel, which enables us to sense our increasing tension. Simultaneously, through these exaggerated actions, we are better able to bring about relaxation.

As was previously noted, anxiety and stress are our body's built-in alarms to alert us to danger. For protection, our body releases hormones that create fight-or-flight responses, and we react appropriately. An unfortunate upshot of anxiety is that it makes us feel insecure, and we begin to question our inner strengths, often leading to a weakening of our coping mechanisms.

In the book *Grateful Brain,* Author Alex Korb said that our brain is conditioned to function in a repeating way. For example, a person who excessively worries about adverse outcomes will subconsciously re-wire his or her brain to process negative information only. Korb noted that our minds cannot focus on positive and negative information at the same time.

By consciously practicing gratitude, we can train the brain to attend selectively to positive emotions and thoughts, therefore reducing anxiety and feelings of apprehension. As with most positive outcomes, gratitude affects the sympathetic nervous system that activates our anxiety responses. At the psychological level, it also conditions the brain to filter the negative thoughts and focus on those that are positive (positivepsychology.com/neuroscience-of-gratitude).

Gratitude activities include a daily journal of the people, places, and things in your life for which you are grateful. When we awake up, and before you go to sleep, express gratitude for the day in whatever way feels comfortable. Consider your own strengths and say them out loud, daily, expressing gratitude for your personal attributes. Share aloud, in a text, email, or phone call, your gratitude to others for who they are and how they have added positively to your life.

My final words on the subject of resilience are that our sympathetic (fight or flight) and parasympathetic (rest or digest) systems do not work in unison. One or the other is dominant. When stress and anxiety are a constant, our bodies are on high and constant alert. All other systems take a back seat, and in some way, they falter. This has become one of my most lengthy chapters because, as I have experienced, it is one of the most crucial for good health. The exciting point here is that in most cases, these factors lie squarely in our control. To conclude, let me say, "Don't worry, be happy!" Your body will thank you for it.

PART 4:
LIVING F.U.L.L.Y.

Aging powerfully is a process that manifests when we fully embrace the fundamentals of a healthy lifestyle, regardless of what we have done to our bodies in the past. The more we become involved in our own physical, emotional and mental welfare, the more vibrant our health will be on an on-going basis, and the more balance we will have in our lives. Our days will be more joyful.

The following precepts of living F.U.L.L.Y. will empower you to move through your years in accord with much of what life has to offer. These behaviors and beliefs will further enrich your years.

F.U.L.L.Y.

F—Fasting

U—Living Unafraid

LL—Laughing and Love

Y—You

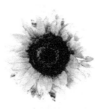

16

THE POWER OF <u>FASTING</u>

Everyone has a doctor in him; we just have to help him in his work.
The natural healing force within each one of us is the greatest
force in getting well….to eat when we are sick is to feed your sickness

~ Hippocrates

Fasting is a natural method of healing.
When animals or savages are sick, they fast.

~ Paramahansa Yogananda

Yes, I said fasting, as in going without food, either for a relatively short period or as long as a month or more. My introduction to fasting was a ten-day stay at True North Health Center, located in Santa Rosa, California, in January 2019, in order to enhance my knowledge and experience a whole food plant-based, SOS (salt, oil, and sugar-free) free diet.

True North, established in 1984 by Drs. Alan Goldhamer and Jennifer Marano, is the largest facility in the world that specializes in medically supervised water-only fasting. My stay there was educational and an induction, if you will. I did not fast, but during my stay I met many people who had remarkable stories of recovery from otherwise intractable illnesses.

The facility houses nearly seventy people, most of whom are safely water fasted for anywhere from 7 to 30 days or longer. If they were not fasting, they were in the re-feeding stage of the process, or like me, were there to learn and enjoy the bounty of fabulous plant based food (although without salt, oil, and fat, it took some getting used to), regenerative rest, health lectures, yoga, cooking classes, and wellness checks.

My affiliation as a health coach at Lifestyle Medical began shortly before my stay at True North, and since then I have participated in five five-day fasts. This fasting protocol is offered at Lifestyle Medical as a supplemental tool to wellness and longevity. In addition, I practice time-restricted feeding (some call it intermittent fasting) on a daily basis. I choose to restrict my daily eating window to approximately 10 hours per day (14 hours fasting), usually from 8:30 am to 6:30 pm. I believe that fasting has been regenerative and one of the smartest things I have done for my health.

Why fasting? Why time-restricted feeding? Dr. Jason Fung, an expert on fasting who is internationally acclaimed for his work in the treatment of diabetes, obesity, and cancer, has based his career on the healing powers of fasting. In his best-selling book, *The Cancer Code,* he suggests that the primary disease pathway of cancer is caused by the dysregulation of insulin, claiming that obesity and type 2 diabetes increase an individual's risk of cancer. One of the strategies outlined in his book is intermittent fasting, which reduces blood glucose and lowers insulin levels. Another is eliminating insulin-stimulating foods, such as sugar and refined carbohydrates.

Dr. Fung, a board-certified nephrologist, explains in another book, *The Obesity Code,* that everything we believe about how to lose weight is wrong, and that weight gain and obesity are driven by hormones. Only by understanding the effects of insulin and insulin resistance can we achieve lasting weight loss. He further explains how intermittent fasting can break the cycle of insulin resistance, allowing us to attain a healthy weight. Dr. Fung offers further insight in yet another book, *Lifestyle in the Fasting Lane: How to Make Intermittent Fasting a Lifestyle.*

My focus on fasting is related to the health benefits. In his YouTube video, The Top 5 Reasons to Fast, Dr. Fung notes some practical benefits that I hadn't considered:

1. Fasting is effective for the treatment of several health risks, including obesity. If you're trying to lose weight, it is powerful because you can't go lower than 0 calories. If you want it to be more effective, fast for longer periods.

2. It can be used in conjunction with any current diet. Whether vegetarian, vegan, Paleo, etc., the only rule is "Don't eat during this period of time."

3. Fasting is free. You can save money in that you don't have to buy anything to make it work.

4. Fasting is convenient. There is no time spent shopping, prepping, or cleaning. It gives time back.

5. Fasting is simple. There are no rules to follow, and it is not complicated. When fasting, don't eat. Doing this forces our body to use its own resources.

Fasting and Longevity

After twenty-five years of comprehensive scientific studies in the lab, the clinic, and among the world's most long-lived populations, Dr. Valter Longo, PhD., has gained a reputation as the international expert on aging. In his bestseller, *The Longevity Diet,* he promotes fasting and claims that periodic fasting can activate stem cells and promote protection, regeneration, and rejuvenation in multiple organs, as well as the nervous system and immune systems. This process significantly reduces the risk of diabetes, cancer, Alzheimer's, and heart disease.

More specifically, he writes, "Periodic fasting promotes stem cell-dependent regeneration in the immune system, nervous system, and pancreas. The fasting itself destroys many damaged cells, and damaged components inside the cells, but activates stem cells. Once refeeding begins, these stem cells become part of a program to regenerate the organ or system with newly regenerated cells bearing characteristics of younger, more functional cells. Additionally, the inside of a variety of cells is partially rebuilt as part of a process called autophagy, also contributing to cellular rejuvenation" (*The Longevity Diet,* V. Longo). This was researched, tested, and proven in both mice and humans.

Dr. Longo goes as far as to recommend a bi-yearly fasting protocol for health and longevity. For those not comfortable with a prolonged water-only fast, he created what he calls a fasting-mimicking diet, a five-day plan that will bring about many of the health parameters of a full fast, but with a calorie-restricted, limited amount of plant-based food that is low in protein and sugar and high in healthy fat. This system was made into a product named ProLon, which I used for my first five-day fast, finding it quite effective. At the Lifestyle Medical clinic, we offer our patients a fasting mimicing option but with an outline of foods (vegetables and nuts or avocado) that they can assemble themselves to create their own fasting-mimicking diet.

Time-restricted feeding (a term Dr. Longo prefers over intermittent fasting) is another component of fasting that he promotes as a daily regime. He is most comfortable with a 10- to 12-hour feeding window, which he believes gives healthy results without potential side effects, one of which is potential gall bladder issues. A twelve-hour feeding window would potentially play out as dinner ending at 7:00 pm, with nothing more to eat until breakfast at 7:00 am. He also discourages eating within three hours of going to bed.

10 Reasons Intermittent Fasting (IF) Is Good for You
(This article was reposted from Authority Nutrition on July 18, 2015)

1. IF changes the function of cells, genes, and hormones. When you fast, insulin levels drop, and the human growth hormone increases. Your cells also initiate important cellular repair processes and change the genes they express.

2. IF can help you lose weight and belly fat by helping you eat fewer calories while boosting metabolism slightly. It is a very effective tool to lose weight and belly fat.

3. IF can reduce insulin resistance, lowering your risk of type 2 diabetes by lowering blood sugar levels, at least in men.

4. IF can reduce oxidative stress and inflammation in the body. This should have benefits against aging and the development of numerous diseases.

5. IF may be beneficial for heart health because studies show that it can improve blood pressure, cholesterol levels, triglycerides, and inflammatory markers.

6. IF induces various cellular repair processes by triggering autophagy, a metabolic pathway that removes waste material from cells.

7. IF may help prevent cancer. It has been shown to help prevent cancer in animal studies and to reduce side effects caused by chemotherapy.

8. IF is good for the brain by possibly increasing the growth of new neurons and protecting the brain from damage.

9. IF may help prevent Alzheimer's Disease. Animal studies suggest that intermittent fasting may be protective against neurodegenerative diseases like Alzheimer's disease.

10. IF may extend your lifespan, helping you live longer. Given the known benefits for metabolism and other health markers, it makes sense that intermittent fasting could help you live a longer and healthier life.

Despite the possible health benefits associated with fasting, it may not be right for everyone. If you suffer from diabetes or low blood sugar, fasting can lead to spikes and crashes in your blood sugar levels, which could be dangerous. It is recommended that you talk to your doctor first if you have any underlying health conditions or are planning a fast for more than 24 hours. Additionally, extended fasting is not generally recommended without medical supervision for older adults, adolescents or people who are underweight.

If you decide to try intermittent fasting, be sure to stay well hydrated and fill your diet with nutrient-dense foods during the eating periods to maximize the potential health benefits. Additionally, if fasting for longer periods, try to minimize intense physical activity and get plenty of rest.

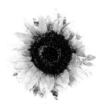

17

THE POWER OF LIVING <u>UNAFRAID</u>

Of all the liars in the world, sometimes the worst are our own fears.

~ Rudyard Kipling

One of the greatest discoveries a man makes, one of his great surprises, is to find he can do what he was afraid he couldn't do.

~ Paramahansa Yogananda

As we age, especially in our later years, it becomes all too easy to look at what we are leaving behind and fear where we are going. At seventy, I am solidly in my later years and have begun to entertain thoughts about "these last few years." It was with this realization that I stomped my foot and said, "No, way. I have at least twenty to thirty years ahead and a purposeful mission with which to fill them!"

Will I live another twenty to thirty years? Who knows?! Will this time be spent remarkably? I don't know that either. But, by dismissing fear and replacing it with anticipation, my outlook has turned around. I committed to writing this book, something I had never done before, uncertain of my ability to do it. I thought I was completely without the skills that one would assume were necessary. But I knew that turning seventy was going to be the beginning of an untested evolutionary period, not the end of something.

Dr. Andrew Huberman, the very popular and accomplished neuroscientist who I mentioned earlier, recently said, "It has been shown repeatedly that attitude follows action." He stressed that when we take action-steps toward whatever we seek to do, enthusiasm and determination will follow. In my case, I looked for a book writing course, enrolled, and began the process. With that, the excitement grew. Was there fear? Yes, at times. But, I kept saying to myself, "You got this, Nan."

As I write, I at times wonder if I will sell even one book. But that isn't the point. By digging up memories that took me to some dark places, I relieved the oppressive weight of them. By putting everything out on the table, I am no longer emotionally constrained by my secrets. By expressing my passion and heartfelt belief in the path to health that has been shown for decades to prevent and reverse our most common chronic illnesses—and which has affected my life in remarkable ways—I have given myself a mission that will carry me through decades. There are no guarantees. But I'm putting fear aside. I'm simply moving forward with purpose and passion.

In his informative, upbeat, and sensitive book, *Not Fade Away: Staying Happy When You're Over 64*, resilience writer Alan Heeks offers guidance to the Baby Boomer generation to enjoy their vintage years and grow through the tough parts of getting old. The book's chapter titles are named after iconic Sixties songs like "Good Vibrations" and "My Generation." The three main sections of his book cover "Finding Your Gifts," "Digging the Challenges," and "Fresh Maps." It's entertaining, insightful and relevant.

In an article for *Living* magazine (September 4, 2018, as outlined on nextavenue.org), Mr. Heeks shares tips from his book:

7 Ways to Beat Your Fear of Aging

1. **Maintain a positive outlook.** The pressures of the world swirling around us may leave us feeling overwhelmed and powerless. We have to continually *choose* to believe in the positives about ourselves, other people, and the world in general. Keep noticing your thoughts and feelings, and keep choosing positive ones, like gratitude and appreciation for all the good things about yourself and life.

2. **Embrace your fears.** Slowing down from the race of our younger years may create space where habitual fears come up more strongly. If you want to grow old happily, my advice is to face these fears of aging sooner, not later. This doesn't mean going into battle with them. Simply invite them to tea and start a dialogue. He explained, "I've found that my fears were just trying to protect me, and they had some useful advice when I gave them a hearing."

3. **Create cheerful daily habits.** Habits are a great way to ensure you keep making the positive choices you need for healthy living. Some examples include continually take time in your day to express gratitude for the good things in your life. Try to bring humor into your daily life by enjoying some comedy on the TV or radio or watching a video. Get outdoors into nature. It will lift your spirits, reduce stress and improve your health. Take a brisk walk, ride a bike, or engage in some outdoor activity every day.

4. **Treat problems as adventures.** Although it is easy to get downcast and feel like a victim when problems in life or health occur, choose instead to believe that there is a gift, an upside to most problems if you can find it. Treat these difficulties the same way you would prepare for an adventure holiday: gather maps and other information, look for a good guide, and treat the new learning you need as an interesting challenge. Look out for any new openings that may arise.

5. **Explore elderhood.** With few guidelines about growing old positively, we have to figure this out for ourselves. He writes, "I'm using the term *elderhood* to invite you to connect to the mature wisdom

in yourself, and in our ancestors." In old tribal cultures, such as the Celts and Native Americans, elders played a vital role in guiding the tribe—to dream dreams, uphold values, mentor the young, and speak truths as they saw them. We live in a very different kind of society today, but the role of the elders is something we can learn from and update.

6. **Be more conscious of your values.** With modern life so hectic and distracting, becoming more aware of your values and choosing to live by them more deliberately can be a real service to your well-being. It's also a gift to those around you, including the younger generation. Values can be everyday ones like honesty, integrity and care for others, as well as choosing to respond positively to the apparently hopeless state of the world.

7. **Cultivate your people skills.** Many research studies show that our ability to express, hear and work with feelings are far more beneficial to our personal and work life than intellect or brainpower. Honing your interpersonal skills is a great step, even for retirees.

Throughout my life, "feeling the fear and doing it anyway," is a mantra that has served me well. This played out most dramatically when my dear husband of 40 years died, leaving the woman who cleaved to him at 18 not sure of who she was at 59. Throwing myself into the unknown, visiting fifteen countries in fifteen months, with everything new and different, challenged me at every turn and brought out a stoicism I didn't know I possessed. Any doubts that I harbored from my early years of feeling unworthy and powerless were quelled when I bravely and capably took on what came to be my greatest challenge, living without the only person in my life who I knew truly loved me, and would always protect me. *Feel the fear and do it anyway.*

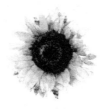

18

THE POWER OF <u>LOVE</u> AND <u>LAUGHTER</u>

Live in the sunshine, swim the sea, drink the wild air.

~ Ralph Waldo Emerson

*Spread love everywhere you go. Let no one ever
come to you without leaving happier.*

~ Mother Theresa

J.D. Salinger, the author of *Catcher in the Rye*, once wrote, "The fact is always obvious much too late, but the most singular difference between happiness and joy is that happiness is a solid, and joy a liquid."

Joy is a stronger and less common feeling among diverse individuals than happiness. Rather than being based in earthly experiences and material objects like happiness, joy is based on spiritual experiences, caring for others, gratitude, and thankfulness. It is inward peace and contentment rather than outward expressions of elation. It is lasting and based on inward circumstances. Joy warms a person's heart while happiness merely pleases; happiness brings pleasure, but joy brings true contentment to one's heart.

The title of this book, *Aging Powerfully: Find Vibrant Health, Balance &*

Joy!, implies a promise. The lifestyle adaptations introduced in this book have been proven to bring about vibrant health and life-balance, both of which I have personally experienced. The goal of this chapter is to introduce ideas and activities that inspire joy.

The secret of a good life may be as simple as one word: *JOY.* When we feel happy and loving, our bodies are flooded with endorphins, our immune system is strengthened, our emotional lives are free of stress and worry, and our relationships improve.

The love I am referring to in this chapter is the type you get when you love yourself, your life, and others. This is different and distinct from the love and strength that we get from others, as I discussed in Chapter 12, *The Power of Others.* It is the feeling that comes from within, and that we then project out to others. This is the love, along with laughter, happiness, and joy, that we create in our own lives and then spread to others.

One of the most dramatic examples of the power of these positive emotions is spotlighted by Kelly Turner, PhD, in *Radical Remission: Surviving Cancer Against All Odds.* Dr. Turner is a researcher and psychotherapist, specializing in integrative oncology. While working with cancer patients, she became intrigued by the instances of complete recovery in spite of dire circumstances and terminal diagnoses.

She invested several years in research, traveling the world, interviewing more than 1,000 recovered patients, as well as various healers, and investigating their remarkable recoveries, which she labeled *radical remissions.* This research later became her PhD dissertation. As I noted earlier, she wrote her book from these documented stories of survival, and while doing so, she noted nine behaviors that all of these patients adopted as part of their personal therapeutic arsenal.

One of her patients, while treating stage 3C ovarian cancer at forty-two years old, succinctly said, "It was clear to me that I would not declare battle but rather find ways to accept and befriend this new and unexpected chapter in my life. I knew that in order to do so, what I needed most was to find gratitude, joy, and fun in life—as often and as much as I was able." In that spirit, she showed up for her first much-dreaded chemotherapy session in purple Converse high tops, explaining, "They made me smile when I walked into that room...those things—joy, fun, kindness and gratitude—that became my true medicine." At the time of this writing, she has been cancer-free for twelve years after multiple recurrences.

Dr. Turner calls laughter, happiness, joy, and love "positive emotions," noting that there is an immediate and powerful connection between the mind and the body and that our emotions create instant bursts of hormones in our brains that tell our bodies what to do. As we have discussed before, negative emotions cause a fight-or-flight response; however, when we feel joy or love, our hormones tell our bodies to spend time repairing broken cells, digesting food, and healing infections. We are either doing one or the other, not both. Therefore, to turn on the health-seeking mode, we must turn off the fight-or-flight mode by making a conscious effort to change our thinking.

In her book, Dr. Turner writes: "We can even escalate this process by *purposefully* trying to feel any number of positive emotions, especially love, joy, and happiness. When we feel these emotions the glands in our brains release a surge of healing hormones into our bloodstreams, including serotonin, relaxin, oxytocin, dopamine, and endorphins, which instantly communicate with all the cells in our bodies, telling them things such as:

- Lower blood pressure, heart rate and cortisol (the stress hormone)

- Improve blood circulation

- Deepen our breathing, which brings more oxygen to each cell

- Digest our food more slowly, which helps the body absorb more nutrients

- Increase white and red blood cell activity, which helps the immune system

- Increase natural killer cell activity, which helps the immune system fight cancer

- Clear out any infection

- Scan for cancer and remove any cancer cells

All of these amazing physical changes have been documented in clinical studies. Similar studies have shown that people who are battling an illness with an overall positive attitude live significantly longer than those people who are pessimistic. In short, happy people live longer!"

Making Joy, Love, Happiness, and Laughter a Habit

While reading the stories of Dr. Turner's triumphant patients, it became clear that they saw happiness as a daily habit, like brushing and flossing. They cultivated the ability to fine-tune and practice this daily in order to reap the desired benefits. They believed that we can *all* experience consistent joy in our lives, as long as we practice feeling happy on a daily basis. This, at times, may mean purposely turning off feelings of fear, discontent, and anger, and replacing them with some joy, even if for only a few minutes.

Activities to increase laughter, joy, and love include:

- Express gratitude daily. Consciously practice this daily.

- Smile and laugh freely, dwell on the positive and don't take yourself too seriously.

- Let forgiveness free you, reclaim a peaceful life that lets your heart sing again.

- Support and serve others. When we give of ourselves in volunteer work, we feel especially fulfilled, energized and good inside.

- Watch a funny movie, YouTube video of animal escapades or anything that makes you laugh.

- Take an energetic or otherwise enjoyable class, such as yoga, Tai Chi, or Zumba.

- Spend time with children, even simply watching them play. Their zeal for life can be contagious.

- Frequent nature and let it astound you. Appreciate the birds and their activities, take in the glory of your surroundings, expand to a panoramic view and fix your gaze on a glorious tree.

- Take time to awaken with a sunrise or end the day with a sunset. Drink it in!

- Create a list of what makes you laugh and check these things off regularly.

- Make a date with play, any kind, that you keep at least once or twice a day.

- Offer your assistance and love to others.

- Join and participate in a positive, upbeat support group.

- Commit to remaining mindful in all you do. Chew slowly and carefully taste your food. Listen well and be present when with another. Be present while doing even minor or repetitive tasks.

- Practice reframing situations in order to see the fun, funny and beneficial aspects of them.

What follows may be a bit technical, but it is a game-changing concept. In his book, *Zen, And the Art of Happiness* (one of my favorite little books), Mr. Chris Prentiss points out that "a key part of our body's incredible communication system involves our cell receptors. Every cell in our body can have millions of receptors on its face, and each cell has perhaps seventy different types of receptors. In the early 1970s, Candace Pert, Ph.D, was the first scientist to prove the existence of these receptors with her discovery of the opiate receptor."

He points out that in her book *The Molecules of Emotion,* Dr. Pert says that "the life of a cell, what it is up to at any moment, is determined by which receptors are on its surface and whether or not those receptors are occupied by ligands, a small molecule that binds itself to a cell receptor. Most are peptides…[or] information molecules that communicate across systems such as neurological, gastrointestinal, and even the immune system. These peptides are produced in the hypothalamus, a gland in the center of the brain, and are *primarily determined by what we think and feel.* The hypothalamus produces peptides that duplicate your experience, from anger, hate, sadness, frustration, and depression, to joy, enthusiasm, contentment, and happiness. These peptides are channeled throughout every cell in our body, dock onto the cells, and create minute physiological phenomena that can translate to large changes in behavior, physical activity, and even mood."

In his film, *What the Bleep Do We Know,* Dr. Joseph Dispenza explains that "when a new cell is produced, it contains more receptors for whatever peptide it received that caused it to split. If the cell received peptides produced by depression, a new cell will have more receptors for depression, and fewer receptors to receive feel-good peptides. Given what we know about peptides, receptors, and the role of emotions and thoughts, you can see the chain of events that take place as new cells are created according to what you think and feel."

"The takeaway from this is that the more you engage in any type of emotion or behavior, the greater your desire for it will become."

Laughter, love, happiness and joy. These emotions are habitual, controllable, and a fundamental part of *Aging Powerfully*. What great news!

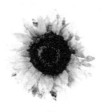

19

THE POWER OF <u>YOU</u>!

*The only person you are destined to become
is the person you decide to be.*

~ Ralph Waldo Emerson

*Be who you are and say what you feel because those who mind
don't matter, and those who matter don't mind.*

~ Bernard M. Baruch

You are special and perfect as you are—worth whatever it takes to make you shine. If you have lost your glow, be true to who you were meant to be. Embrace your weaknesses, your quirks, your brilliance, your sense of style, your individuality, and your possibilities. Play it up!

Perhaps these words are easier to say than to internalize. Having turned seventy-years young, a life lesson that I hold dearly is that in the end, we create our own experience. Through the law of attraction, we bring about what we think about. Aging powerfully embodies accepting our past, living our best life moving forward, and putting into place what that represents for us. YOU are at the core of a most excellent adventure from here forward. Below you will find thought-starters to help you crystalize your vision of YOU:

1. Take time to answer these questions: Who am I? What do I really want? They are existential questions but easy to digest. Begin by looking at who you are by making a list of your greatest strengths and any desires you have to build on them. Then look at what more you want in life, and take note of how you are already on your way. Your goal is to applaud who and what you are, and to have a destination you can embrace. Don't confuse old values with new ones; we are moving forward here, and in many cases with new insights.

2. Be confident. Become self-aware and strengthen your consciousness. Know what makes you feel good and what doesn't. Then construct the habits of doing what makes you better and avoiding what makes you worse.

3. Take time to list what you are good at and passionate about. Honor yourself by marrying the two, be it a hobby you adopt, a class or certification program you undertake, or a new venture that you launch. Let your special light shine.

4. Your previous choices and behavior, although impactful, do not define who you are, nor need they affect who you are transitioning into as you age more powerfully every day. Stay steadfastly fixed on who you are and on where you are going from this day forward.

5. Focus on change and growth with the eyes of a child. Try new things and take on challenging tasks, repeating to yourself the whole while, "I GOT THIS!" Get a little wild. Wear your sequins with your high-top tennis shoes. Let yourself be unpredictable and a bit mysterious. The point is to let a part of yourself shine that you may heretofore have kept shrouded.

6. The things you say to yourself matter. What you think about yourself will result in your becoming that person. Use your mind to frame your thoughts in a positive way. Make it a daily habit of catching yourself doing something right. Take a bow and applaud yourself.

7. Believe strongly in yourself and never give up. Regardless of where you came from, how you were treated, or how you treated yourself, see the star that you are. Hold your head high, and put your shoul-

ders back. When you look in the mirror, see all of the beauty there is and the unique attributes that constitute your glow. Be your own best friend and your own hero.

8. Let a part, or all, of your wardrobe take on a persona of its own. Craft it to make a statement about you, one that resonates with who you know you are now. Show it off to the world.

9. Do the same with a corner of your home. Make it a special space that embodies a side of yourself that isn't always on display but that the world should know about. Express your glorious individuality.

10. Recognize that life is only what you make of it. Why not make it magical, wonderful, beautiful, and maybe even a little strange. In some way, do something every day that thrills you. Tap into your deepest best self, let that shine, and express yourself.

11. Embrace your POWER! Trust who you are and what you were put on this earth to accomplish. Let your essence well up inside of you and fearlessly, enthusiastically, and joyously move toward a clear vision of how you want to grow from here. Carry the banner in your special way and encourage those around you to make the choice to AGE POWERFULLY.

Here's to YOU!

I will finish this book and this chapter with a focus on *you*. You hold your future in your hands. My exhaustive research, time with patients, and clear evidence among those who live by the lifestyle recommendations outlined in this book have fueled my passion for spreading the word: you can control how you age. By making simple lifestyle changes, you can add years to your life and life to your years. In some cases, these adaptations may mean making changes to ingrained habits, but I promise you that these changes will become second nature and then preferential. What you add to your life becomes a far greater satisfaction than what you give up. It may take time, but it will happen.

There is a joke going around—something to do with a man telling his doctor that if he had to give up the long list of things that are killing him, he would just as soon die. It's not very funny when those very things he isn't willing to reject kill him slowly and tortuously. His body parts begin to erode, procedures begin to mount up, and life becomes a physical slog.

The right lifestyle choices can allow us the full use of our physical and mental faculties well into our nineties and beyond. I like to think of my own diligent lifestyle choices as my way of "squaring the curve." What curve, you ask? It is the downward curved line from good health to ultimate death that begins for most Americans in their fifties and ends in their mid-seventies (the current average American life expectancy for a man is 76.7, and for a woman, it is 81. Note that it has dropped in each of the past three years. Chronic diseases (80% of which are lifestyle-related) take hold and modify our bodies, stealing life from us. My goal at seventy is to relish the idea of another twenty to thirty years of vibrant health, balance, and joy—to live like those in the Blue Zones who enjoy active and happy lives until they die. The process at the end is then relatively quick. In other words, live till you die, rather than live, break down, suffer, decline, and then die. These are harsh words for an even more harsh reality.

I will leave you with heartfelt best wishes to take control of your health. Live your life focused on a long and joyous outcome. And whatever you do, make it your mission to *AGE POWERFULLY!*

JOIN THE MOVEMENT

Grow old along with me!

The best is yet to be.

The last of life, for which the first was made:

Our times are in His hand

Who saith "A whole I planned,

Youth shows but half; trust God: see all,

Nor be afraid!"

~ Robert Browning
taken from his dramatic monologue "Rabbi Ben Ezra" (1864)

Grow old along with me! The best is yet to be. There is no denying that whatever path we take, age will have a say on our life; let's seek the joy and not be afraid.

Join me in celebrating this third and final act of my life. There is so much more to say about this mission of ours to age powerfully. Visit my website, join my newsletter, and reach out to me on Facebook and Instagram. Let's form a community of people committed to showing what AGING P.O.W.E.R.F.U.L.L.Y. looks like!

Email: AgingPowerfully@gmail.com

Website: www.NanSimonsen.com

Instagram: www.instagram.com/agingpowerfullywithnan

Facebook: www.facebook.com/agingpowerfullywithnan

RESOURCES: READING, WATCHING AND LEARNING

Books

General Plant Base Nutrition and General Health

Fiber Fueled: The Plant Based Gut Health Program for Losing Weight, Restoring You Health, and Optimizing Your Microbiome by Will Bulsiewicz, MD, MSCI. Includes recipes.

The Blue Zones: 9 Lessons for Living Longer from People Who've Lived the Longest by Dan Buettner

Reversing Diabetes: The Scientifically Proven System for Reversing Diabetes Without Drugs by Dr. Neal D. Barnard, MD. Founder and President of the Physicians Committee for Responsible Medicine. Includes recipes.

Your Body in Balance: The New Science of Food, Hormones, and Health by Neal D. Barnard, MD, FACC. Includes recipes.

The Vegan Starter Kit: Everything You Need to Know About Plant-Based Eating by Neal D. Barnard, MD, FACC. Includes recipes.

The OMD Plan: Swap One Meal A Day to Save Your Health and Save the Planet by Suzy Amis Cameron. Includes récipes.

The China Study: The Most Comprehensive Study of Nutrition Ever Conducted by T. Coli Campbell, PhD and Thomas M. Campbell II, MD. Startling implications for diet, weight loss, and long-term health. Founded the T. Colin Center for Nutritional Studies

Whole: Rethinking the Science of Nutrition by T. Colin Campbell, PhD

The Secrets to Ultimate Weight Loss: A Revolutionary Approach to Conquer Cravings, Overcome Food Addiction, and Lose Weight Without Going Hungry, by Chef AJ, with Glen Merzer. Includes recipes.

Unprocessed: How to Achieve Vibrant Health and Your Ideal Weight by Chef AJ. Includes recipes.

Own Your Health: How to Live Long and Avoid Chronic Illness by Glen Merzer. With over 75 delicious, nutritious recipes by Chef AJ

The Microbiome Solution: The Radical New Way to Heal Your Body from the Inside Out by Robynne Chutkan MD, FASGE. Founder of the Digestive Center for Women. Includes recipes.

Forks Over Knives: The Plant-Based Way to Health. The How-To Companion to the Landmark Documentary *FORKS OVER KNIVES.* Includes recipes.

Eat To Live: The Amazing Nutrient-Rich Program for Fast and Sustained Weight Loss by Joel Fuhrman, MD. Includes recipes.

Prevent and Reverse Heart Disease: The Revolutionary, Scientifically Proven, Nutrition-Based Cure by Caldwell B. Esselstyn, Jr., MD. The book behind Bill Clinton's life-changing plant-based diet. Includes recipes.

Plant-Strong: Discover the Worlds Healthiest Diet, With 150 New Engine 2 Recipes by Rip Esselstyn

How Not to Die: Discover the Foods Scientifically Proven to Prevent and Reverse Disease by Michael Greger, MD

How Not to Diet: The Groundbreaking Science of Healthy, Permanent Weight Loss by Michael Greger, MD, FACLM. Founder of nutritionfacts.org

The Starch Solution: Eat the Foods You Love, Regain Your Health, and Lose the Weight for Good by John A McDougall, MD. Includes recipes.

The Longevity Diet: Discover the New Science Behind Stem Cell Activation and Regeneration to Slow Aging, Fight Disease, and Optimize Weight by Valter Longo, PhD. Director of The Longevity Institute, USC

Not Fade Away: Staying Happy When You're Over 64!: The baby boomer guide to creative aging by Alan Heeks

The Vegiterranean Diet: The New and Improved Mediterranean Eating Plan—With Deliciously Satisfying Vegan Recipes for Optimal Health by Julieanna Hever, MS, RD. Includes recipes.

Food Rules: An Eater's Manual by Michael Pollan

In Defense of Food: An Eater's Manifesto by Michael Pollan

UnDo It!: How Simple Lifestyle Changes Can Reverse Most Chronic Diseases by Dean Ornish, MD, and Anne Ornish. Cofounder of the College of Lifestyle Medicine and founder and president of the nonprofit Preventive Medicine Research Institute. Includes recipes.

Eat More, Weigh Less: Dr. Dean Ornish's Life Choice Program for Losing Weight Safely While Eating Abundantly by Dean Ornish, MD

Diet for a New America: How Your Food Choices Affect Your Health, Your Happiness, and the Future of Life on Earth by John Robbins

The Food Revolution: How Your Diet Can Help Save Your Life and Our World by John Robbins

The Plantpower Way: Whole Food Plant-Based Recipes and Guidance for the Whole Family by Rich Roll. Includes recipes.

The Alzheimer's Solution: A Breakthrough Program to Prevent and Reverse The Symptoms of Cognitive Decline at Every Age by Dean & Ayesha Sherzai, MD, codirectors of the Brain Health and Alzheimer's Prevention Program at Loma Linda University Medical Center. Includes Recipes.

Cookbooks

The Blue Zones Kitchen: 100 Recipes to Live to 100 by Dan Buettner

The China Study Cookbook by LeAnne Campbell, PhD

The China Study All-Star Collection by LeAnne Campbell, PhD

The Kick Diabetes Cookbook: An Action Plan and Recipes for Defeating Diabetes by Brenda Davis, Rd and Vesanto Melina, MS, RD

The Prevent and Reverse Heart Disease Cookbook: Over 125 Delicious, Life-Changing, Plant Based Recipes by Ann Crile Esselstyn and Jane Esselstyn

The Engine 2 Cookbook: More Thank 130 Lip-Smacking, Rib-Sticking, Body-Slimming Recipes to Live Plant-Strong by Rip Esselstyn and Jane Esselstyn

Eat To Live Quick & Easy Cookbook: 131 Delicious Recipes for Fast and Sustainable Weight Loss, Reversing Disease, and Lifelong Health by Joel Fuhrman, MD

The How Not to Die Cookbook: 100+ Recipes to Help Prevent and Reverse Disease by Michael Greger, MD, FACLM

Vegan Richa's Indian Kitchen: Traditional and Creative Recipes for the Home Cook by Richa Hingle

Eat Vegan on $4.00 a Day: A Game Plan for the Budget Conscious Cook by Ellen Jaffe Jones

Ageless Vegan: The Secret to Living a Long and Healthy Plant-Based Life by Tracye McQuirter, MPH with Mary McQuirter

Vegan Under Pressure: Perfect Vegan Meals Made Quick and Easy in Your Pressure Cooker by Jill Nussinow, MS, RDN

The Kind Diet: A Simple Guide to Feeling Great, Losing Weight, and Saving the Planet by Alicia Silverstone

Forks Over Knives, The Cookbook: Over 300 Recipes for Plant Based Eating All Through the Year, by Del Sroufe

Recovery Related Books

Breaking the Food Seduction: The Hidden Reasons Behind Food Cravings— And 7 Steps to End Them Naturally by Neal Barnard

The Cheese Trap: How Breaking a Surprising Addiction Will Help You Lose Weight, Gain Energy, and Get Healthy by Neal Barnard

Brain Over Binge: Why I Was Bulimic, Why Conventional Therapy Didn't Work, and How I Recovered for Good by Kathryn Hansen. One woman's story gives binge eaters hope, a new perspective, and a commonsense cure.

The Brain Over Binge Recovery Guide: A Simple and Personalized Plan for Ending Bulimia and Binge Eating Disorder by Kathryn Hansen

Starving In Search of Me: A coming-of-Age Story of Overcoming an Eating Disorder and Finding Self-Acceptance by Marissa Larocca

The Pleasure Trap: Mastering the Hidden Force that Undermines Health & Happiness by Douglas J. Lisle, PhD, and Alan Goldhammer, DC

Radical Remission: Surviving Cancer Against All Odds by Kelly A. Turner. The 9 key factors that can make a real difference

Rational Recovery: The New Cure for Substance Addiction by Jack Trimpey

Additional Reads

Radiation Nation: Fallout of Modern Technology, Your Complete Guide to EMF Protection & Safety by Daniel T. DeBaun and Ryan P DeBaun

Wherever You Go There You Are: Mindfulness Meditation in Everyday Life by Jon Kabat-Zinn

Clean My Space: The Secret to Cleaning Better, Faster—and loving your home every day by Melissa Maker. Founder of cleanmyspace.com

Documentaries/TV

Eating You Alive

Forks Over Knives

The Game Changers

What the Health

Cowspiracy

Years of Living Dangerously

Websites

The National Eating Disorders Association: www.nationaleatingdisorders.org

The National Association of Anorexia Nervosa and Associated Disorders: www.anad.org

National Suicide Prevention Lifeline: suicidepreventionlifeline.org
800-273-8255

Binge Eating Disorder Association (BEDA): www.bedaonline.com

Environmental Working Group: www.ewg.org

American College of Lifestyle Medicine: www.lifestylemedicine.org

Forks Over Knives: www.forksoverknives.com

NutritionalFacts.org (Dr. Michael Greger): nutritionfacts.org

Physician's Committee for Responsible Medicine (Dr. Neal Barnard): www.pcrm.org and www.pcrm.org/health/diets/kickstart

eCornell Plant based certification program: eCornell.com

Institue for Integrative Nutrition online health coach courses: Integrativenutrition.com

Nan's EMF meter:

TriField Meter Model 100XE
Reads magnetic, electric, and radio/microwave